Office Surgery
for Family Physicians

Office Surgery for Family Physicians

WALTER J. PORIES, M.D.
FRANCIS T. THOMAS, M.D.

Department of Surgery
East Carolina University
Greenville, NC

BUTTERWORTH PUBLISHERS
Boston • London
Sydney • Wellington • Durban • Toronto

Chapters 4, 9, 10, 13, 17, 21, and 23 were illustrated by Carol J. Pienta. Chapter 18 was illustrated by Tamara Bell and Carol J. Pienta. Chapters 11, 12, 16, and 25 were illustrated by Rebecca A. Dodson. Chapters 7, 19, and 24 were illustrated by Charles W. Kesler. Chapter 22 was illustrated by Rebecca A. Dodson and Carol J. Pienta.

Every effort has been made to ensure that the drug dosage schedules within this text are accurate and conform to standards accepted at time of publication. However, as treatment recommendations vary in the light of continuing research and clinical experience, the reader is advised to verify drug dosage schedules herein with information found on product information sheets. This is especially true in cases of new or infrequently used drugs.

Library of Congress Cataloging in Publication Data

Pories, Walter J.
  Office surgery for family physicians.

  Includes index.
  1. Surgery, Outpatient.   I. Thomas, Francis T.
II. Title.   [DNLM: 1. Ambulatory Surgery.
WO 192 P8360]
RD110.P67 1984   617'.91   84–12040
ISBN 0–409–95142–0

Butterworth Publishers
80 Montvale Avenue
Stoneham, MA 02180

10 9 8 7 6 5 4 3 2 1

Printed in the United States of America

This book is dedicated to our wives, Drs. Mary Ann Rose and Judy Thomas, both excellent scholars, who have, through their dedication to research, service, and education, inspired our careers.

Contributing Authors

Byron Burlingham, Ph.D.
Professor and Chairman
Department of Microbiology
East Carolina University
Greenville, NC   27834

Paul S. Camnitz, M.D.
Associate Clinical Professor
Department of Surgery
Division of Otorhinolaryngology
East Carolina University
Greenville, NC   27834

Ed Janosko, M.D.
Assistant Clinical Professor
Department of Surgery
Division of Urology
East Carolina University
Greenville, NC   27834

Walter J. Pories, M.D.
Professor and Chairman
Department of Surgery
East Carolina University
Greenville, NC   27834

Francis T. Thomas, M.D.
Professor of Surgery
Department of Surgery
East Carolina University
Greenville, NC   27834

Steven M. White, M.D.
Clinical Professor and Chief
Department of Surgery
Division of Ophthalmology
East Carolina University
Greenville, NC   27834

Contents

Contents

Contents

Preface

The purpose of this book is to provide primary care physicians an amply illustrated guide for managing two kinds of surgical problems encountered in ambulatory office practice: "minor" surgical problems and emergency procedures.

"Minor" surgical problems include those such as the treatment of paronychiae, lacerations, and thrombosed hemorrhoids, as well as the performance of biopsies. The text describes those types of surgical procedures, which, under certain constraints, can be properly and safely performed in an office setting by skilled family physicians, pediatricians, internists, emergency room personnel, and the resident staffs in those specialties.

This book also contains vital information on emergency procedures, ranging from chest tube insertion or establishing an airway to complete cardiopulmonary resuscitation, which the primary care physicians may be called upon to perform in a life-threatening emergency. It is a ready reference to guide the emergency support until the patient can be transferred to a major medical facility. The prepared primary care physician is still the first line of defense in most parts of the United States; he or she is frequently the first (and often the only) doctor to reach a moribund patient in time to institute effective emergency therapy.

The limitations and potential dangers of office surgery are well known and carefully set out in this book. Within these limitations, office surgery performed by the patient's primary care physician has outstanding potential. For the patient, it often represents the least amount of inconvenience, travel time, emotional upset, and cost. These are the precise reasons why the patient chooses his primary care physician under most circumstances of illness. From the primary care doctor's point of view, he or she can give more complete care, provide better and easier follow-up, and achieve these important goals at minimal cost.

In discussing office surgery with colleagues, we found surprising agreement among surgeons that:

1. since many of these procedures are already being handled in primary care offices, they ought to be dealt with in the most current and effective manner;

2. unfortunate delays, in such diseases as breast cancer, for example, can be avoided if the initial needle aspiration biopsy is done at the first doctor contact; and

3. lancing boils, evacuating paronychiae, and performing needle biopsies, although an appropriate part of a surgeon's armamentarium, are not the most effective use of a highly trained surgeon's time.

We have a personal feeling that underlies all of the precepts of this book: surgery is the art and science of a physician caring for a patient using techniques that have come to be called "surgical." Surgery is not magic, though it may seem so to the patient; it is not "minor" and is never viewed as such by the patient or the understanding physician. It can be performed by family physicians, just as drugs can be dispensed by surgeons, and it is a precious and costly human activity that should be done by a qualified doctor under conditions that are of optimal benefit to the patient primarily and society secondarily. This book examines a small part of surgery and helps to delineate more clearly the role of the family doctor in office surgery.

We want to express our deepest gratitude to our many co-workers who gave invaluable help to the writing of this book. In particular, we would like to thank Tammy Bell, Rebecca Dodson, Maureen Fox, Charles Kesler, Ellen McGowan, Carol Pienta, Betsy White, Robin Williams, and Wayne Williams for their important help. We are also extremely grateful to Arthur Evans, Kathy Benn, and the staff of Butterworth Publishers for their help in getting the final draft into publication expediently.

Walter J. Pories, M.D.
Francis T. Thomas, M.D.

Foreword

We are fortunately entering an era when it is fashionable for physicians to strive to keep patients out of the hospital for many medical and surgical procedures. The cost of hospital care and concurrent public impatience with the escalating cost of receiving health care in acute care hospitals have led to several alternatives to hospital admissions for surgery. The widespread establishment of quick-in/quick-out surgical centers in many communities in the United States underscores the need for re-examining the issues involved in ambulatory surgery. This book could not have been published at a more appropriate time in the evolution of modern medicine.

Whether the apparent relationship between the emergence of family medicine as an established specialty and the national trend toward an increased emphasis on ambulatory health care is one of cause and effect is a question best left to the rhetoric of medical politics. The fact remains that many family physicians and their patients find it increasingly desirable to perform many surgical procedures in the office setting. This excellent book provides a ready reference for the family physician in the performance of office surgery and for the management of life-threatening surgical emergencies.

An accomplished and successful artist in his own right, Dr. Pories has effectively used the old adage, "A picture is worth a thousand words." I found that he has very appropriately used diagrams and pictures for clear communication of the details of surgical techniques and has also provided a method of teaching office personnel. The focus of the content is on the ordinary more than the extraordinary, the common more than the rare.

Although there is wide disparity within the specialty of family medicine regarding the extent of surgery performed in that practice in various regions of the country, the authors have written this book for family physicians who include office surgery as a part of their armamentarium. It is intended to be an atlas for family physicians engaged in the practice of office surgery and is not meant to replace the standard text oriented toward major hospital-based surgery.

Finally, the book is a strong statement by a highly respected surgeon that it is appropriate for family physicians to perform those ambulatory surgical procedures for which they have been properly trained. As a colleague of Dr. Pories for many years, I can speak to his support of family practice. On numerous occasions I have heard him begin his lecture to a new class of medical students by saying, "A surgeon is a family doctor who performs surgery." I am sure this book will be widely read and reread by family physicians in both practice and academic settings. Walter Pories is a unique professor of surgery, and his book deserves to be included in the library of every family physician interested in office surgery.

James G. Jones, M.D.
Professor and Chairman
Department of Family Medicine
East Carolina University

Chief of Staff
Department of Family Practice
Greenville, NC

Vice President of
American Board of
Family Practice Physicians

I · General Principles

1 · *Outpatient Surgery*

FRANCIS T. THOMAS, M.D.

Outpatient surgery is the oldest form of surgery. For centuries, surgery was (and sometimes still is) performed in the patient's home, the doctor's office, or a makeshift facility at the site where the patient was injured or incapacitated. Surgical instruments were few, and anesthesia consisted only of alcohol or such narcotics as opium, given by mouth. Only after the development of anesthesia in the 1840s did hospital facilities become the site of most major surgical procedures.

Recently, in an effort to lower costs and improve health care, a revival of outpatient, office, or ambulatory surgery has taken place. At present, approximately 20% of all primary patient-surgeon contacts in the United States occur in the outpatient department. Moreover, recent experience with outpatient facilities suggests that 30% to 40% of all surgery could be performed in an outpatient facility, a potentially sweeping cost-cutting reform. So-called ambulatory surgery performed in a unit associated with a hospital complex is, however, rarely as cost-effective or convenient for the patient as surgery in a free-standing ambulatory unit (surgical center, or Surgi-Center), and in fact, the individual practitioner's office in many respects offers the greatest cost-effectiveness and patient convenience. The prototype of the free-standing surgical ambulatory facility, the Surgi-Center established in 1970 in Phoenix, Arizona, has accommodated more than 50,000 procedures without a single operative mortality. Although the family practitioner may find some of the arrangements of the surgery center unsuitable for office surgery, he can learn much from studying such a facility.

Almost any procedure that does not invade the abdominal, thoracic, or cranial cavities may be considered for outpatient surgery. In addition, some operations within the colonic cavities, such as laparoscopy, tubal ligation, hernia repairs in children, and insertion of chest tubes for drainage, can be done well in a modern surgical center. These operations are, of course, too extensive for office surgery, but they are mentioned to demonstrate how much can be done on an ambulatory basis. The procedure must be relatively minor, however, and the anesthesia required must also be such that the patient can recover sufficiently to return home shortly after the operation.

Very few physicians in office practice currently undertake general anesthesia in the course of their practice. Dentists have used general anesthesia in the office fairly extensively, but most have now supplanted this practice with the use of local anesthesia and nerve blocks, which, in combination, can produce safe and profound anesthesia. Perhaps the single factor most responsible for curtailment of general anesthesia in the office has been the increase in malpractice cases, threatening costly judgments against the practitioner who has an unfortunate accident (usually a cardiac arrest) during office administration of general anesthesia.

Spinal or epidural anesthesia is usually unsatisfactory for office procedures because it produces temporary lower-extremity paralysis, which interferes with the patient's locomotion, and it may also cause hypotension from spinal vasodilatation.

Of the most common surgical procedures such as abscess drainage, skin lump excision, hemorrhoidectomy, vasectomy, procedures through the sigmoidoscope, and plastic surgery, perhaps 25 to 30% can be performed in the office, and 40 to 50% might well be done in a free-standing surgical facility. Office surgery will always have some limitations that do not pertain to free-standing surgical facilities of the Surgi-Center type. Such a free-standing facility can maintain a full complement of equipment and personnel for general anesthesia, cardiopulmonary resuscitation, and the extensive surgical procedures necessary for controlling bleeding and similar complications. Although the family practitioner can use office surgery to tremendous advantage, he or she must be wary of performing complication-ridden procedures too extensive for safe performance in the office setting.

While office surgery is very safe in general, tragic and costly medical malpractice suits have been associated with minor surgery performed in a nonhospital facility. Although such surgery is perceived by the patient and family as being minor and therefore uncomplicated, all surgery has potential for dire complications. The malpractice issue as it concerns office surgery is also complicated by the fact that courts tend to rule against practitioners of office surgery, posing the persuasive question: Why was this surgery not performed in a better-equipped and better-staffed facility? The prudent family practitioner will accept for office surgery only those cases unlikely to produce complications that would require more extensive facilities or personnel for control.

The overall cost of outpatient surgery is about 50 to 70% less than that for inpatient surgery. Third-party carriers, recognizing this fact, are offering incentives to encourage office, ambulatory, or outpatient surgery, and in some cases they are increasing physicians' remuneration for outpatient surgery over inpatient surgery.

Another important advantage of outpatient surgery is involvement of the patient and family in health care. One of the major failures of our health system has been its inability to impress upon the patient the need for participation in his or her health care.

Outpatient surgery involves the patient and family much more directly in care than inpatient surgery, where more of the care is performed by medical personnel. The patient and his or her family have responsibility at home for both proper preoperative preparation and postoperative aftercare. All family members thus must come to a rather full understanding of the patient's disease and care. They have the advantage of being able to keep the patient more comfortable than other, unfamiliar, caretakers could. Although the family practitioner encourages family involvement in most instances, the way in which the family is involved may be dictated or limited by the family practitioner. Certain family members may lack the compassion and common sense so important in caring for the patient, while others who are skillful in this area can be brought more directly into patient care. It is up to the physician to explore such arrangements in detail, providing clear direction.

The practitioner of outpatient surgery must ensure that the patient is safe for the surgery and that the surgery is safe for the patient. Outpatient surgery is not a good idea for unreliable, uncooperative, or unintelligent patients likely to disregard or fail to understand instructions. Such patients may come to surgery unprepared and fail to follow instructions given them for home care after surgery, with possible unfortunate or even disastrous consequences.

PSYCHOLOGICAL CONSIDERATIONS

Although we discuss this subject more completely in another chapter, a word needs to be said concerning the psychology of outpatient surgery. The patient undergoing outpatient surgery is normally anxious, anticipating a completely new experience. Rarely does any patient feel that any surgery happening to him or her is minor. Outpatient surgery at best involves a high level of anxiety and some pain. Proper premedication and anesthesia are therefore essential. Whenever you inflict pain upon a patient, regardless of the patient's understanding, he or she perceives such pain as a visceral reaction of unpleasantness. While the patient's cerebral cortex may be saying, "This is an orderly and necessary procedure," his or her lower brain centers are saying, "Damn, that hurts." In many instances, patients make no bones about the fact that you have hurt them and that they are unhappy. One cannot overemphasize the importance of premedication, alleviation of anxiety, and anesthesia adequate to reduce or eliminate pain during the surgical procedure.

The surgeon's demeanor is also important to the level of patient anxiety. A doctor who is profusely sweating, clearly unnerved, speaking in anxious tones to his assistants, and operating with a shaking hand will do little to allay the observant patient's anxieties. It is important to operate calmly, with quiet deliberation. Sometimes it may be necessary to stop for a moment to allay the patient's anxiety; one should always explain to the patient what is about to happen at each stage of surgery but avoid unnecessary or frivolous conversation.

There are some interesting differences between major inpatient surgery with the patient under general anesthesia and outpatient surgery. In terms of the doctor's demeanor, outpatient surgery is the more demanding. When the patient is under general anesthesia, slips of the tongue, the hand, the foot, and any number of embarrassing mistakes remain unknown to the oblivious patient. In contrast, in outpatient surgery, the patient is usually wide awake and fully aware of the surgeon's actions. Remarks patients sometimes make after an outpatient procedure under local anesthesia make one realize the great need for unbroken professional demeanor. Casual comments about the progress of the surgery, often made unconsciously by the surgeon during intense concentration, can be quite upsetting to patients.

Another source of annoyance to patients is the well-meaning but talkative medical assistant given to inappropriate and unnerving remarks, which can be easily misinterpreted by the anxious patient.

FACILITY AND EQUIPMENT

Outpatient surgery can be performed in a room as small as 10 × 10 ft, although a more commodious room, such as 15 × 15 ft or even 20 × 20 ft, allows more equipment in the operative area.

The room should be relatively secluded to keep traffic, contamination, and noise level down. There is nothing more unnerving for doctor or patient than traffic or noise in the operative area. The room itself should be pleasant, painted a soft but cheerful color, suggesting comfort and warmth. Cold objects such as surgical instruments, surgical lighting fixtures, and other medical equipment should be kept in closed cupboards and drawers whenever possible.

The most important piece of equipment is the examining and operating table; it should have a full complement of electrically operated devices for raising and lowering, tilting, and breaking (bending by angles) at the appropriate spots for the patient to assume a supine, prone, jackknife, semi-Fowler position, and so on with the least inconvenience. Many patients undergoing outpatient surgery are uncomfortable or in pain; any movement of these patients will be met with unhappiness. The newer tables permit minimal movement of the patient to achieve the positions required for treatment. These newer tables, attractive and warm in appearance, are made more comfortable by the soft cushions provided.

Such tables provide good exposure of all areas of the body except the upper extremities. Providing an advantageous, comfortable working area for upper-extremity surgery can be difficult. Some tables are provided with arm-board attachments, usually the most satisfactory means of exposing lesions of the upper extremity for inspection, diagnosis, or surgery. Some lesions of the distal extremity can be treated by bending the elbow and bringing the arm across to rest on the patient's chest or abdomen. This is usually an unsatisfactory position for a variety of reasons, however, and we recommend extension of the arm onto an arm board for most upper-extremity incisions. The arm board should allow rotation of the extremity to a position above the plane of the patient's head or below the plane of the patient's lower abdomen, to allow proper cleansing and aseptic preparation of the surgical site. An assistant is sometimes needed to hold the hand in the air until the aseptic preparation can be performed; the hand or arm can then be lowered onto sterile towels placed over the arm board. Such a job should not be relegated to a weak medical assistant. A strong assistant, if one is available, for moving patients onto a table and positioning them for surgery is a great help to the doctor and a comfort to the patient.

Lighting is an essential aspect of office surgery. The surgery room should contain a wall-mounted light source accommodating a photoscope, ophthalmoscope, and a lamp mounted on a plastic band to fit around the surgeon's head. Such a headlamp is by far the best source of light for suturing deep lacerations or for good illumination in a difficult area. The traditional gooseneck lamp, so familiar to all of us, is not satisfactory; it provides poor light, obstructs the surgical field, and is a source of heat and discomfort for both patient and surgeon. At least one and preferably two overhead room lights with good mobility, along with high-efficiency fluorescent lights, are desirable for adequate overall illumination for surgery. Floor-mounted lamps adjust poorly to the angles required for illuminating the depth of some wounds and have many other disadvantages. The operating headlamp is an inexpensive substitute if overhead lighting cannot be provided.

The surgical room should have a sink and surgical soap for the physician's scrub, as well as for preliminary washing of dirty instruments prior to sterilization. In my opinion, the ordinary sink with hand faucets is preferable for outpatient surgery, but a surgical sink with foot control for turning water on or off does permit more thorough cleansing for the physician and the assistants. The physician should wash his or her hands thoroughly and frequently, especially in the patient's presence. Patients will often comment about a physician's not washing his or her hands before or after contact with them.

SURGICAL INSTRUMENTS

A complete and diversified supply of surgical instruments should be available for office surgery. Maintaining such an inventory requires a considerable effort; a conscientious and skilled person should be assigned the job of developing and maintaining the surgical equipment, in cooperation with the surgeon. There is no ideal inventory; the selection must be individualized for each practitioner and the requirements of his or her practice. Practitioners differ widely in their preferences for surgical instruments and suture materials. All too often, the practitioner relegates selection of this equipment to a nurse, then complains about the type of equipment and sutures purchased. This very important matter should be attended to personally by the individual practitioner.

The surgical instruments are best kept in small sterile multipurpose packs. At our institution, we include the following items in each of the packs:

- 12 4-×-4-in gauze sponges

- 2 medicine glasses

- 1 pair bone forceps

- 2 pairs curved hemostats

- 2 pairs straight hemostats

- 1 knife blade holder

- 1 pair needle holders

- 4 forceps

- 2 retractors

- 1 pair iris scissors

- 2 pairs 4-in straight scissors

- 1 pair 5-in straight scissors

- 1 pair 4-in curved scissors

- 2 folded green towels

- 2 towel clips

- 1 curved medicine bowl scissors

- 1 blunt-tipped probe

In addition, we keep a variety of instruments available in separate wrappers:

- 4 curved mosquito clamps

- 4 curved Crile clamps

- 2 Vanderbilt clamps

- 2 Kelly clamps

- 2 pairs iris scissors

- 2 pairs curved Metzenbaum scissors

- 2 pairs Mayo scissors

- 2 crochet hooks

SUTURES, DRAINS, AND DRESSINGS

- Nonabsorbable suture
  Prolene: 2-0, 3-0, 4-0, 5-0 with tapered needles; 3-0, 4-0, 5-0 with cutting edge needles

- Absorbable suture
  Vicryl ties: 2-0, 3-0, 4-0; Vicryl: 2-0, 3-0, 4-0, 5-0 with tapered needles; 4-0 with cutting edge needles
  PDS: 1-0, 2-0, 3-0 with tapered needles

- Paper Steri-strips: 1/4 in, 1/2 in

- Skin stapler (disposable), staple removers (disposable)

- Catheters
  Salem sump: #16, #18 French
  Malecot: #10–20 French
  Red rubber: #6–20 French

- Drains
  Penrose: 1/4, 1/2, 1 in
  Jackson-Pratt suction catheter with reservoir

- Dressings
  2- × -2-in, 4- × -4-in gauze squares
  Q-tips
  Cotton balls
  Kerlix and Kling bandages
  Elastic bandages
  2-, 3-, 4-, 6-inch plaster rolls and splints

- Dressing medications
  Vaseline gauze
  Betadine gauze
  Neosporin ointment
  Tincture of benzoin

THE CRASH CART

A crash cart containing basic life-support equipment including an Ambu bag, airways, endotracheal tubes, laryngoscope, intravenous (IV) fluids, infusion sets, needles and IV catheter, blood pressure cuff, and appropriate medications should always be in the room or immediately available and easily accessible.

We have found that the tool cart offered by Sears is an excellent crash cart because it is inexpensive, easily moved, and can be locked. The upper drawers hold the following items to serve as an acute resuscitation tray.

Pharmacy

- Nitroglycerin (5 vials)
- Sodium bicarbonate (10 vials)
- Epinephrine 1:10,000 (5 vials)
- Epinephrine 1:10,000 with cardiac needle
- Lidocaine 100 mg (5 vials)
- Lidocaine 1 gm (5 vials)
- Atropine (5 1-mg vials)
- Calcium gluconate (5 1-gm vials)
- Isuprel 1:5,000 (2)
- Dopamine (Intropine) (2)
- Dextrose 50% (5 50-gm vials)
- Valium (10-mg syringe)
- Sterile saline (5 300-cc bottles)
- Sodium chloride (5 500-cc IV bottles)
- 5% dextrose in water (5 500-cc IV bottles)

Respiratory Therapy

- 2 oxygen tanks with gauze and volume regulator
- 2 connecting tubing O_2
- 2 O_2 cannulas
- 1 O_2 catheter
- 1 O_2 mask (pediatric)
- 2 aerosol adapters
- 1 pediatric cannula
- 1 pediatric mask
- Ambu (positive pressure ventilating) mask and bag with oxygen connector
- Suction machine or wall outlet
- 1 Yankauer suction top and tubing
- Suction catheters, disposable, for endotracheal suction

Intravenous Equipment

- #14, 16, 18, and 20 Angiocath (plastic catheter over needle)
- #14–26 plastic intravenous lines with attached needles
- Tourniquet and alcohol sponges
- Tape for securing intravenous lines
- Three-way stopcock and 5 10-cc syringes

Cardiopulmonary Resuscitation

- Cardiac direct current (DC) defibrillator with oscilloscope monitor and paper EKG

- Laryngoscope and endotracheal tubes sized from 2 to 8 mm

Endoscopy Equipment

- Otoscope

- Ophthalmoscope

- Sigmoidoscope
Large sigmoidoscopy swabs
Biopsy forceps to fit through sigmoidoscope

Cautery

- Small portable unit (Hyfrecator type)

The office surgery room should also contain a microscope, a hemocounter, stains for the examination of smears for organisms and to permit differential counts of white cells, and a chamber for the counting of white cells. A small centrifuge is needed to measure the hematocrit and to examine urinary sediments and wound discharges. Many of these tests can be done in the office while the physician or the assistant is taking the patient's history, at great savings to the patient.

The surgery room's medicine cabinet should contain agents for treatment of seizures and any epileptic responses, local anesthesia conduction blocks, and premedication. A partial list of such agents would include a short-acting barbiturate such as sodium pentobarbital (Nembutal), 1 and 2% lidocaine (Xylocaine) with and without epinephrine, diazepam (Valium), morphine sulfate, epinephrine solution (1:1,000), diphenylhydantoin (Dilantin), and intravenous procaine for treating cardiac arrhythmias. Adverse reactions from local anesthetic agents require immediate countermeasures; thus, medication must be at hand for treatment.

The surgery room must be well equipped. The absence of adequate resources from a minor surgery room can be and often is grounds for malpractice litigation in the event of an adverse occurrence during minor surgery.

2 · *Legal Aspects of Outpatient Surgery*

FRANCIS T. THOMAS, M.D.

The steadily increasing trend of elective surgery done in outpatient facilities brings with it increasingly complex medicolegal concerns. Although surgical operations done in outpatient facilities are usually minor procedures, there is ample opportunity for medical malpractice actions to arise from such surgery. A familiar example is the so-called anesthesia mishap. In a healthy person undergoing local anesthesia for a minor elective procedure, cardiorespiratory dysfunction, anoxia, or both may occur, with resultant permanent brain damage. If such an event were to befall a very sick person hospitalized in an acute care facility and undergoing surgery for a life-threatening condition, a jury would be likely to be understanding of the many risks attending such a situation; a physician charged with malfeasance in that case would be likely to receive a favorable judgment. In the outpatient situation, however, where the patient is often young, clearly healthy, and undergoing a minor and elective procedure, an anesthesia death is hard for a jury to understand. In such a case, a judgment will likely go against the surgeon and involve a huge sum of money.

In seeming paradox, those surgical specialties in which most of the cases involve minor elective outpatient surgery carry the highest premium for medical malpractice insurance, while cardiovascular surgeons, for example, who repeatedly perform high-risk surgery on very sick patients, have much lower rates for malpractice insurance.

Observation of certain fundamental principles greatly reduces a surgeon's likelihood of being sued for medical malpractice. They are not complicated or esoteric. In fact, obedience to these principles constitutes nothing more than good medicine, but they are too often honored in the breach.

Compassion is of paramount importance. Many malpractice suits originate in a poor relationship between patient and doctor or patient's family and doctor. The surgeon may be perceived as haughty, dispassionate, unsympathetic, or frankly incompetent. The best possible professional and emotional relationship with patient and family is the surest insurance against a malpractice action. In the climate of such a relationship, patients often overlook physician error. No surgeon will ever achieve the desired result in every single case, even under the best of circumstances, but a carefully nurtured doctor-patient relationship usually predisposes the patient to overlook any shortcoming.

Competence in patient care is also of critical importance. Patients today value and demand a high degree of technical competence in their surgeons, and judges and jurors are very knowledgeable and usually capable of objectively evaluating competence. The operating room, heretofore a mysterious inner sanctum, is today commonplace on the television screen, with all its intricacies and complexities clearly described. Recent surveys indicate that the public is far more interested in a physician's competence than in his or her personality. Modern physicians have a wealth of high-technology diagnostic and therapeutic tools at their command. They should make every effort to inform themselves about their best use.

Deliberate, clear, *preoperative explanation of the surgery, its aims, and the risks involved* is essential. Many malpractice suits stem from disagreement between patient and physician as to whether the patient was fully informed of the possible aftereffects or dangers of the therapy. *Informed consent* is a term heard frequently today; the most common malpractice action involving informed consent is brought by a patient who feels he or she was not apprised of the nature of the therapy, the goals the surgeon hoped to accomplish, or the risks involved in a procedure. The average patient approaches surgery with a high level of emotion; it is understandable that a brief explanation can be misunderstood. Use of complicated medical terms adds to the confusion. A consent form should be worded as simply as possible, in language understandable by a layperson of average or less than average education, and the physician's explanation should be expanded by use of clear diagrams and illustrations when possible.

The surgeon should have *clear documentation that the consent form was obtained.* The form should state in specific terms the nature of the therapy and the potential risks and possible undesirable effects of such therapy, the patient should sign the form and date it, and signatures of witnesses should be clearly appended as well. A completed consent form must be present in the medical record before any surgery is begun.

The surgeon must be the leader of the health care team, regulating the competence of all ancillary personnel in the surgical suite, but he or she must also demonstrate a charitable understanding of any member of the team whose action may lead to unfortunate consequences, provided it is an isolated event and not a habitual one. A surgeon who is willing to admit and take responsibility for his or her errors will earn the respect of the other members of the team; he or she will be all the more respected if he or she demonstrates a willingness to support and strengthen the self-esteem of any member of the surgical team who makes a single unfortunate mistake. Building loyalty in this way will produce the teamwork and willingness to give the extra effort necessary for the very best patient care. Sympathetic understanding of any unavoidable misadventure in the operating room must go hand in hand with every precaution to prevent its habitual occurrence.

PERSONAL LIABILITY AND HEALTH CARE PROVIDER LIABILITY

Under U.S. jurisprudence, corporate health care providers, including hospital outpatient clinics and similar facilities, may be held accountable for medical malpractice. Outpatient surgeons must understand their responsibility within the facilities where they work if they are to protect themselves against potential malpractice suits. In fact, surgeons may carry double liability if they should be stockholders of the outpatient facilities in which they work. Any staff member of an institution providing health care should inform him- or herself of the institution's standards for outpatient care and mechanisms for correcting excesses or defects. Some states require free-standing facilities such as outpatient surgical centers to maintain codes for their facilities and to furnish to the patients a description of their rights and the facility's responsibilities. Such a statement must declare who advised the patient of his or her rights, the proposed course of treatment, the prospects for recovery, and the identity of the person or persons directly responsible for the patient's care.

Outpatient surgery center codes also include a statement of the patient's responsibilities in relation to the facility. These include the following:

- Keeping appointments and promptly informing the physician by telephone or other prompt communication of any complications;

- Following the recommendations and treatment prescribed by the physician, including taking medications and following instructions pre- and postoperatively;

- Indicating to the physician at any time if the patient seems not to understand the prescribed form of therapy or the goal and objectives;

- Providing a complete and accurate medical history including any severe reactions to drugs, allergies, and other conditions that might seriously injure the patient's health if not disclosed to the physician. In the latter regard, *it is extremely important for the physician to document clearly and accurately any failure of the patient to discharge these responsibilities.* Unless this is done immediately, it is highly unlikely that a patient will later admit a shortcoming on his or her part, and a physician will have trouble convincing a judge or jury that his or her retrospective testimony is accurate.

The courts are increasingly recognizing that the patient-physician relationship involves duties and responsibilities on both sides. In many cases, courts have ruled that it was clearly a patient's responsibility rather than a physician's for abandoning a particular form of therapy, with injurious effects. In the early postoperative period after outpatient surgery, there is heavy responsibility on the patient and family, in contrast to inpatient surgery; for, once the patient has been discharged from the facility, responsibility for prompt reporting of complications, proper postoperative care, and monitoring of the patient no longer lies with hospital personnel. Hemorrhage or other grave postoperative complications, if not promptly observed and reported to the physician, can be a catastrophe; the same applies if a patient cannot be transported to the physician promptly enough for treatment of such a complication. Many lawsuits have charged the surgeon with being unavailable or failing to respond to an urgent call for a postoperative complication.

The free-standing surgical center appears particularly vulnerable in this regard, in contrast to the acute care facility, which maintains a number of house staff and other paramedical personnel to respond to emergencies. Surgeons who divide their time between acute care facilities and outpatient facilities may also be vulnerable to charges of negligence because they often come to rely on the availability of skilled physicians in the acute care facility and forget that there is no such back-up on-call group in the outpatient facility.

Outpatient center surgery thus calls for faultless communication in all directions—surgeon to staff, surgeon to patient, patient to staff, patient to surgeon, staff to surgeon, staff to patient—if trouble is to be avoided.

CONCLUSION

Adherence to the principles outlined in this chapter will defuse most of the potential for malpractice litigation associated with outpatient surgery. Patient responsibility for follow-up and prompt notification of the physician of any problems merits repeated emphasis. Surgeons should state clearly to patients their role in the relationship; a patient information booklet is a good way to provide this message. Outpatient surgeons must make certain they are amply covered with back-up care and faultless communications systems. Prudence in this regard will eliminate many problems. The best back-up system is one that will uncover a problem as early as possible, alert the surgeon promptly to the difficulty, and allow an early remedy.

3 · Pain Control

FRANCIS T. THOMAS, M.D.

Pain is the most common complaint of patients seeking the aid of a physician and is probably the aspect of disease that worries the patient most. The patient and practitioner often approach the matter in different ways, with the practitioner's primary focus being the disease process, prognosis, and treatment and the patient's concern being the ravages of disease such as disability and pain.

Office surgery, of necessity, carries some potential for pain before, during, and after the surgery. The patient may seek surgical relief for a painful lesion such as an abscess. Injections of a local anesthetic agent or other anesthetic manipulations often cause pain. During most office surgical procedures, there is a constant potential for intraoperative pain. Finally, the pa-

tient will feel pain at the surgical site for hours to days following the procedure.

We can summarize some general principles about pain. Pain is the awareness of a reaction that begins in visceral or somatic nerves. Somatic nerve sensation is concentrated primarily in the skin and subcutaneous tissues, although all structures of the integument, including muscle and bone, are capable of pain sensation. Visceral pain, coming from the peritoneum, pleura, or other structures lining body cavities, is different from somatic pain in that it is felt more deeply in the body, is often difficult for the patient to localize, and may be duller and more diffuse than somatic pain. Visceral pain may result from distention of an innervated structure, whereas somatic pain is usually produced by inflammation or trauma to a particular structure. Some structures in the visceral cavity, such as deep layers of gallbladder, liver, spleen, kidneys, and other organs, are essentially devoid of pain nerve fibers and become painful only when a surrounding capsule or a lining structure becomes inflamed or stretched. Visceral pain especially and, sometimes, somatic pain are associated with a spectrum of unpleasant sensations including a sense of ill-being, anorexia, nausea and vomiting, or other severe symptoms. Severe visceral pain is one of the most unpleasant sensations known; a person experiencing this type of pain is usually fearful in the extreme of recurrence of the pain.

In addition to its physiological component, pain clearly has a strong psychic component. This relationship is important to the practitioner primarily for two reasons. First, because of the strong psychic elements in pain, the practitioner can often predict the degree of pain that will accompany a given procedure through knowledge of the patient's psyche. Second, reduction or alleviation of a patient's anxiety about a surgical procedure often does much to reduce the severity of pain felt by the patient. Clear and direct communication between patient and physician may allay any fear of the unknown; a habitually cheerful and competent air on the practitioner's part in his or her communications with the patient will also serve this end.

An equally important psychic factor bearing upon pain perception is the fact that pain often brings a patient face to face with intimations of his or her mortality and serves as a reminder of the presence of the disease process. Pain may be so all-pervasive that it causes the patient to focus exclusively on the pain and the disease process, so that other areas of the patient's life not related to the disease often become sublimated to the pain and its attendant emotional reaction. In the grip of severe pain, the strongest of men and women will become angry, act irrationally toward the practitioner and other health care professionals, and exhibit near-psychotic behavior.

Somatic and visceral pain impulses must pass through a number of neural circuits before they are perceived in the cerebral cortex as sensations. The pain can be interrupted by any of various therapeutic techniques: a direct block or severance (either temporary or permanent) of the involved sensory nerve, such as a nerve block and local infiltration; the use of drugs to control pain at various levels; and the use of drugs to reduce or allay anxiety.

Throughout the ages, humans have used medical, religious, and even mechanical means for dealing with pain. In some societies today, one still can witness the use of primitive (and often effective) means of handling pain. The technique of acupuncture, for example, has been passed down through the ages. Little is known of its mechanism of action, but it is certainly effective in handling some types of pain, although its principles seem blatantly unscientific at times. Some drugs used for pain, such as morphine and its derivatives and alcohol, have been widely known for their analgesic effect for many centuries. Indeed, both minor and major surgery (such as amputations and even abdominal operations) of centuries past were performed with only morphine and alcohol (and sometimes only one of the two) to control pain. A major advance in temporary local pain control was the use of cocaine as a local anesthetic agent, by Sigmund Freud and others. Subsequently, many surgeons applied local anesthetic techniques, finding them the only satisfactory alternative to the very dangerous technique of general anesthesia using chloroform and ether.

Local anesthesia and nerve blocks are the mainstay of office surgery today and have been greatly expanded in scope by a large variety of agents and techniques, described in Chapter 6. These agents act by interrupting the nervous circuit at the site of their injection into the nerve or in the nearby structures with subsequent neural infiltration. The action of local anesthetic agents can be prolonged and enhanced by mixing them with epinephrine, which causes vasoconstriction and thus slows absorption and migration of the local anesthetic agent.

Local anesthetic agents such as lidocaine can completely block pain from the local nerves for hours; they remain the best and safest of the anesthesia techniques. The anesthesia techniques commonly used in office surgery are discussed in Chapter 6.

General anesthesia characterizes the techniques for relieving pain. With any of these techniques the patient loses consciousness, ranging from mild sedation to deep unconsciousness. General anesthesia renders the patient oblivious to pain and trauma, but it has two great disadvantages: (1) various complications can develop, and (2) complex equipment is necessary for its proper administration and monitoring. General anesthesia is not recommended for most office surgery.

Pain control before, during, and after office surgery has much to do with surgical success. Most frequently overlooked is postoperative control of pain; patients are often sent home without proper analgesia. Left to their own means, these patients often become confused and agitated because of their pain and discomfort; the practitioner may be unavailable or the patient may not know whether to call him or her. "I thought the pain would get better and I didn't want to bother you, doctor," is a frequent response. The patient's family may feel great sympathy for his or her suffering and often harbor anger toward and dissatisfaction with the practitioner in such an event. In my view, ample analgesia is necessary for at least two to three days after any office surgery or until the next office visit; the patient should understand clearly how to reach the physician and the arrangement by which more pain medication is available, if necessary. Caution is advised, however, because some patients abuse analgesics, and others seem to require far more medication than the surgical procedure seems to warrant.

Pain can be a very misleading symptom and may be attributed by the physician to the wrong cause. It seems natural after any surgical procedure to view any lingering pain as a sequela of the surgery. However, the practitioner must be constantly wondering whether the pain is coming from another source.

Pain at the site of surgery can usually be alleviated by rest, elevation of the part, supportive bandaging, or splinting. Occasionally, an ice bag (for lacerations associated with sprains) or warm compresses (following the drainage of abscesses) will give relief. If the pain is excessive, the patient should be seen as quickly as possible, and the wound must be totally undressed and inspected. Dangerous causes of pain include a constricting dressing or cast, an expanding hematoma, and infections such as tetanus, gas gangrene, symbiotic gangrene, erysipelas, and fasciitis.

Various analgesic medications are available to the practitioner; they act to relieve pain by one of several mechanisms. Some agents reduce inflammation, a common cause of pain at the site of surgery or trauma. Inflammation at a surgical site is a normal, positive bodily defense mechanism and should not normally be impeded.

However, inflammation at the site of trauma, especially nonpenetrating trauma such as a muscle injury or a sprain, can often be controlled by one or another of the many anti-inflammatory compounds available. Recent physiological studies have shown that virtually all anti-inflammatory compounds, including steroids, inhibit the release and activity of a variety of agents in the prostaglandin pathway. Prostaglandins are ubiquitous compounds that initiate or amplify inflammatory response in an area of infection or trauma. Steroids act at the cellular level to prevent the release of arachnodonic acid compounds, which serve as the basis for prostaglandin synthesis and prostaglandin-induced inflammatory reactions. The so-called nonsteroidal anti-inflammatory agents [including aspirin, phenylbutazone (Butazolidin), ibuprofen (Motrin), zomepirac sodium (Zomax), indomethacin, and many other compounds] also inhibit prostaglandin synthesis and block prostaglandin pathways. Thus, in using any of these drugs, the practitioner is accomplishing a rather similar biopharmacologic effect but not to the same degree. Steroids are potent anti-inflammatory compounds, effecting the most powerful anti-inflammatory responses that can be induced pharmacologically. They are also associated with various undesirable effects, and even the short-term use of such agents entails the risks of promoting sepsis and other potentially dangerous conditions. Aspirin, in contrast, one of the mildest anti-inflammatory agents, often is not very effective in its anti-inflammatory action. Some of the newer nonsteroidal anti-inflammatory agents are fairly potent and can be useful for the office practitioner in the control of inflammatory pain. Again, we should point out, however, that agents interfering with the inflammatory response are often inappropriate or contraindicated in office surgery, especially if an incision or penetrating trauma is involved. Some specific nonsteroidal anti-inflammatory agents and their dosage are as follows: zomepirac sodium, 100 mg q 4–6 h prn; ibuprofen, 300–600 mg 3 or 4 times a day; phenylbutazone, begin with 300–600 mg/day in 3 to 4 divided doses, maximum therapeutic effects can usually be obtained with 400 mg daily in divided doses. Leukopenia and gastric symptoms are serious side effects that require dose monitoring.

Opiates have long been an important adjunct to the medical management of pain. Opiates are narcotic analgesics, natural or synthetic, similar to derivatives of opium. Morphine and codeine are two of the more important of the 20-odd alkaloids in this family. Meperidine hydrochloride (Demerol) is perhaps the most widely used analgesic agent in hospital practice. Opiates produce various undesirable effects including somnolence, depression of respiration, stimulation of the nervous system (in some instances producing nausea and vomiting), and responses from virtually all body systems. Careful questioning of the patient and family is wise; a history of allergic response to the opiates is not uncommon.

The opiates have a marked analgesic effect and greatly reduce painful sensations for those patients who can take them. The most common effects felt by a patient given a strong therapeutic postoperative dose of an opiate-derivative analgesic include euphoria, drowsiness, and sometimes (especially with morphine) nausea and vomiting. Meperidine hydrochloride is preferred over morphine because of the far lower incidence of nausea and vomiting and because it is available as an oral preparation. Parenthetically, morphine can be given orally for severe pain and is used widely as an elixir (15 mg/tsp) for terminally ill patients. Two-thirds is absorbed, making 15 mg given orally equivalent to 10 mg given subcutaneously. The opiates produce analgesia lasting from a few hours up to a day. Over 90% of a dose of morphine or meperidine hydrochloride is excreted within 18 to 24 hr in most people; the usual frequency of administration is about every 3 hr as needed; continuous analgesia is desired for moderately uncomfortable pain. The usual dose of morphine, 5 to 10 mg, is far more effective when given frequently. The usual dose of meperidine hydrochloride, 50 to 75 mg, is usually more rapidly effective than morphine. For oral analgesia, codeine is perhaps the best drug of all. The usual dose is 15 to 30 mg given every 4 to 8 hr. Pentazocine (Talwin) is a drug with moderate effects. In higher doses it may produce bizarre behavior and is not usually a very effective analgesic. Tolerance for and physical dependence on pentazocine do occur.

The intravenous administration of low-dose opiates during the procedure is useful in difficult cases and usually produces no lowering of blood pressure (a very important advantage of these agents in general anesthesia). Meperidine hydrochloride can depress respiration, however, and if it is used in the office, one of the opiate antagonists such as naloxone hydrochloride (Narcan) should be available to counteract respiratory depression.

The broad classification of tranquilizing sedative drugs is useful in reducing preoperative anxiety and for intraoperative sedation. The most popular and useful are diazepam (Valium) and the barbiturates sodium pentobarbital (Nembutal) and phenobarbital. Although these agents cause drowsiness and some euphoria and usually reduce anxiety, they are poor analgesics and will not produce sufficient analgesia for even the most minor office surgical procedures. They often help to relieve postoperative pain by reducing anxiety and thus reduce the amount or potency of the required analgesics. Recent studies demonstrate that diazepam, like the barbiturates, causes both a physical and psychological dependence. Prolonged use of this agent and of the barbiturates may cause drug dependence; therefore, use of both diazepam and the barbiturates should be confined to the immediate postoperative period. The usual dose of diazepam is 5 to 10 mg q 3 to 8 h prn. The patient needs to be warned that this drug can cause drowsiness and disorientation and that these side effects are synergized by alcohol consumption. The usual dose of barbiturates is 50 to 100 mg. These agents are most frequently given as a single dose preoperatively but may be used postoperatively in controlling anxiety. The barbiturates cause drowsiness and chemical dependency, and the practitioner is wise to avoid chronic administration to a patient for any purpose.

Drugs in the phenothiazine family and other psychotropic agents such as rauwolfia have largely fallen into disuse in outpatient surgery. Such drugs are poor analgesics and have a wide variety of psychotropic effects (usually weak ones). Although their use in management of severe neuroses and psychoses seems established, the office practitioner will find little use for these drugs in the management of perioperative anxiety.

Phenothiazine drugs, often referred to as major tranquilizers, or antidepressant agents are often used to treat chronic pain syndromes in family practice. In office surgery they have little use, however, since they provide no analgesic effect. The phenothiazines and antidepressants do have specific uses in some unusual pain syndromes, always chronic and often associated with psychic changes. Such syndromes are rare, producing very unusual effects, and should be treated by specialists in neurology or neurosurgery.

We have recently been impressed with the small, battery-operated, portable electric stimulators that are attached to the patient's skin with adhesive terminals. The degree of electric stimulation can be adjusted by the patient. In about half of our small series, these devices have produced considerable comfort. They are especially useful in patients with metastatic disease.

In summary, good pain control for office surgery begins with minimization of preoperative anxiety by communication and education when possible and by the use of tranquilizers when anxiety reduction is not possible. For a patient who comes to the office with severe pain from trauma, an analgesic such as an opiate derivative may also be given. The practitioner must make an accurate diagnosis, identifying the true cause of the pain. Local anesthesia by direct injection or nerve block is the most effective and safe technique for pain control. After surgery, patients should have some type of analgesic agent appropriate to the magnitude of the surgery and trauma and a means of obtaining additional analgesics or tranquilizers for the first two to three postoperative days. Use of analgesics, tranquilizers, or other such drugs for relief of pain from office surgery for more than a week is unwise. Thorough familiarity with a few drugs and repetitive use of them is better than the infrequent use of a multiplicity of drugs. Each drug has advantages and disadvantages, and each produces particular effects of which the practitioner must be aware, guarding against undesirable effects or overdosage. Effective control of pain prior to, during, and following office surgery will perhaps do as much as anything to produce patient satisfaction.

4 · *Manual Skills and Surgical Tools*

WALTER J. PORIES, M.D.

Surgical technique is not difficult to learn, but it does take practice. The few basic manipulations—cutting, clamping, grasping, tying, and sewing—are not inherently difficult to master. The physician who has learned these basic skills enjoys office surgery rather than dreads it. The rewards are also great; patients do better and their wounds heal nicely with minimal scars.

Practice is worthwhile. Just as a musician practices before a concert, and a professional basketball player shoots practice baskets, the physician can refine surgical skills on materials easily obtainable at the local market. Fruits, broiler chickens, and pigs' feet are excellent materials for practicing surgical techniques. In our surgery course for medical students, we ask them to excise letters, numbers, and imaginary lesions from grapefruit with scalpels; the broilers and pigs' feet are excellent for learning dissection and closures. It is surprising how quickly a smooth technique can be developed in such a stress-free setting.

CUTTING

Tissues should be cut cleanly and perpendicular to their surfaces for optimal healing:

Skin is best incised with a scalpel. The tissue should be stretched until taut, and the blade should be held at a 90-degree angle to the surface of the skin for a clean cut.

1

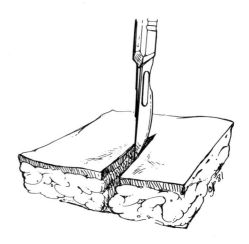

Hesitation, loosely held skin, and an angled scalpel produce jagged wounds that heal imperfectly with wide, ugly scars.

2

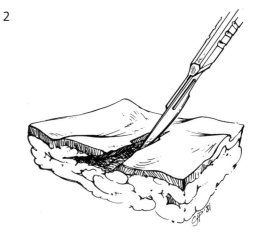

Incisions heal better if they are made parallel to wrinkle lines and across the lines of muscle pull. Such wounds frequently approximate themselves; exercise and activity actually aid in keeping the wound edges together.

3

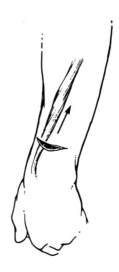

The wrinkle lines are easily demonstrated by gently pinching the skin and subcutaneous tissues. The pinching is done from several directions; the ideal incision line is indicated where the wrinkles form most easily with minimum pressure.

4

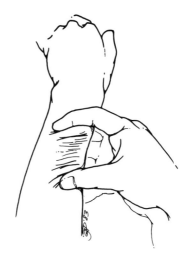

Scalpels come in a variety of shapes and sizes. For most office procedures, however, a #15 blade mounted on a #3 handle will serve nicely.

5

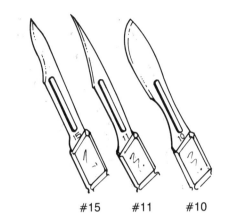

#15   #11   #10

For the fine work required for office surgery, the scalpel is best held like a pen or pencil. The classic underhand, four-finger grip useful for long abdominal or chest incisions does not allow the precision required for small incisions and excisions.

6

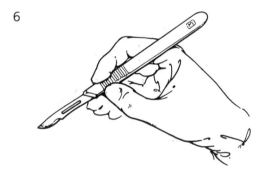

Scissors are by far the best tool for cutting and dissecting the deeper tissues under the skin. Scissors are versatile because they can be used closed as a dissector, can separate tissue planes bloodlessly by their spreading action, and provide better control and greater safety than scalpels during the dissection or excision of lesions.

Scissors come in a variety of designs. For the office, the delicately curved Metzenbaum and the more heavily curved Mayo scissors will serve for most problems; occasionally, small iris scissors will prove useful. Blunt points are easier to handle and serve nicely to push tissues; sharp points are seldom needed in office practice. Although it is traditional to use straight scissors to cut sutures, the curved scissors are equally effective. It is not really necessary to buy an extra set of straight scissors just to cut thread.

7

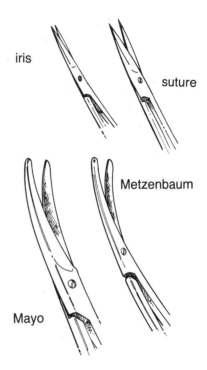

iris

suture

Metzenbaum

Mayo

Scissors (and clamps) are best held with the thumb and ring finger pushed only partly into the rings of the instruments (a). If the fingers are inserted fully, action is sharply hampered and release is difficult. The index finger stabilizes the scissors or clamp from above, and the ring finger provides stability from the side (b). The grip deserves practice because it allows maximum spread of the jaws and solid control.

8a

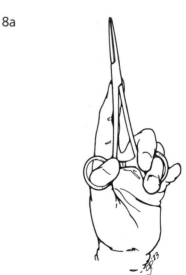

8b

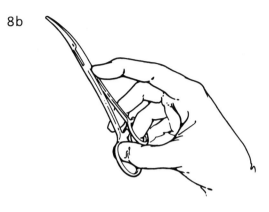

When scissors are used for dissection, the tips
should be inserted into the tissue plane, the
curve of the instrument being aligned with the
shape of the tissues being excised. Gentle
spreading of the jaws defines the plane and
usually divides the thin areolar tissues, leaving
the stouter strands that may contain small vessels, nerves, or other structures. These strands
can then be cut cautiously; if they contain vessels, the spreading allows them to be defined
more easily so they then can be clamped or
cauterized before they are cut.

9

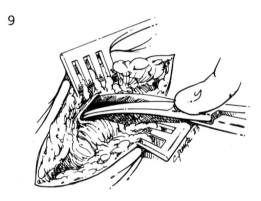

Because scissors cut by crushing, in contrast to
the clean incision of the scalpel, they are not
normally used for cutting skin. Dull scissors or
dull scalpels are dangerous. They should be
sharpened or discarded.

CLAMPING

Office surgery should be almost bloodless; that is, the operative field should be dry so that the tissue planes can be easily seen, there is no hematoma to retard healing, and the patient is not frightened by his or her hemorrhage.

A dry field is obtained by judicious and precise clamping of blood vessels that can then be divided and ligated or cauterized without blood loss. Accordingly, the clamp should be used only to grasp vessels precisely, without including extraneous tissue. Clamps crush and kill tissues; if they are not used with precision, they can cause much damage and seriously interfere with healing.

Clamps best grasp the individual vessel preferably with the concave side of the instrument toward the tissues. Grasping tissues *en masse* with the convex side toward the wound not only damages tissue but also may frequently fail to include the bleeding vessel.

Clamping should be performed deliberately; it is never necessary to rush. No matter how large the vessel, bleeding can always be controlled initially by pressure. The vessel can then be exposed slowly and clamped as it appears. It is useful to remember the old surgical adage, "Clamp the vessel, not the stream."

Clamps should not be used to hold specimens being excised. This practice fragments delicate tissues such as lymph nodes and may crush them to the extent that they are unfit for microscopic examination.

Small bleeders can occasionally be controlled by the so-called clamp-and-twist method. After the bleeding vessel has been isolated and clamped precisely, the clamp is twisted three times about its own axis. Although the technique is not as dependable as ligature or cauterization, it can be helpful if assistance or a cautery is not available.

10

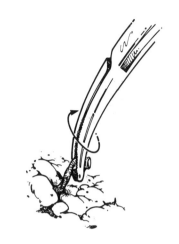

Ligature

The most secure method for the control of a bleeding vessel is the clamp-and-ligature technique. The bleeding artery or vein is first grasped with a fine clamp, which is then used to lift the vessel so that a fine ligature (3-0 or 4-0) can be placed (a) and tied below the clamp (b). It is important that the ligature not pull the vessel up from the tissues because small arteries or veins are easily severed, especially if the tissues are inflamed and therefore friable. The ligature should be tightened by keeping the knot stable and pulling the ends against each other rather than against the vessel. The clamp is removed just as the knot is tightened down to minimize the chance of the suture's cutting through the vessel. Two additional knots are then placed to secure the knot. Although it is traditional to tie a square knot with the second knot, it is often better to tie a granny initially so that the knot can be tightened just a bit more. A third knot is then applied to make the square.

11a

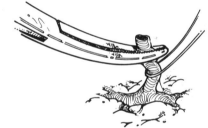

11b

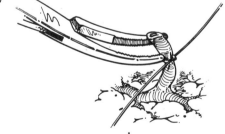

Double Ligature

Occasionally, where an unusually large or difficult bleeder is encountered, extra security may be required. The double-clamp, double-ligature approach answers this need. Two clamps are placed on the bleeding vessel, and the first tie is placed below both clamps (a). The lower clamp is then removed (b), and a second tie is placed above the first (c). The technique has the advantage of retaining control of the vessel during the entire application of the first knot and is therefore also a useful method if one is working with an untrained assistant.

12a

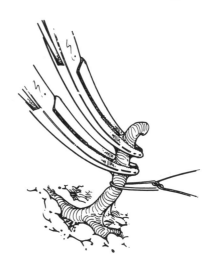

12b

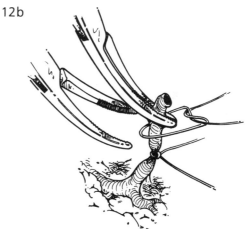

12c

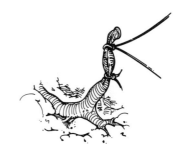

Ligature in Continuity

This method is rarely needed in office surgery but can be most useful in the care of traumatic emergencies. The vessel is dissected gently from the surrounding tissues so that the two sutures can be tied about 1 cm apart. When these are secure, the vessel is then divided.

13c

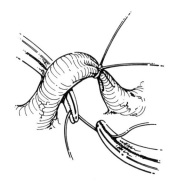

13a

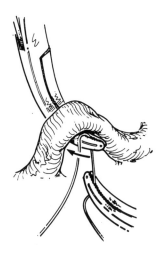

13d

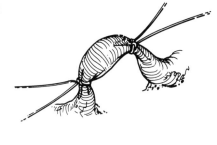

13b

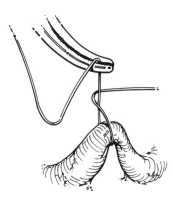

13e

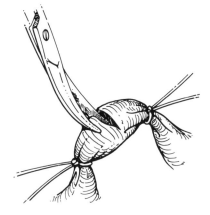

Additional control can be obtained by adding a suture ligature on the flow side of the vessel, as illustrated.

14a

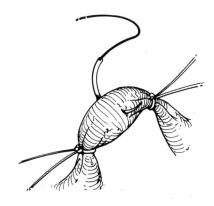

14b

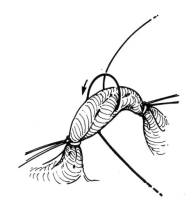

14c

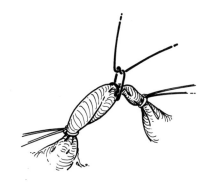

Cautery

The cautery is a useful tool in office surgery. A brief touch to the clamp controls the clamped vessel, eliminating the need for ties and, frequently, for an assistant as well. We feel that the cautery is now a must during office surgery because it affords such a margin of safety, simplifying procedures that were previously difficult and time-consuming because of excessive bleeding. We have been pleased with the Hyfrecator, but models by other manufacturers may serve equally well.

15

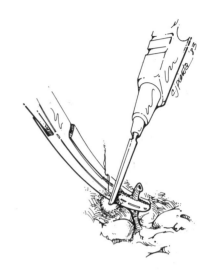

GRASPING

Grasping is usually done with forceps. The forceps should be precise, gentle enough to permit delicate handling of the tissues, and fitted with fine teeth so that only minimal pressure is necessary to grasp the tissue without crushing.

Forceps come in a large variety of designs, but two types should meet all of the requirements of office surgery: the fine-toothed small Adson forceps and the larger but still delicate DeBakey forceps. The smooth forceps should be avoided because they crush tissues and require considerable pressure to keep tissues in their grasp.

16

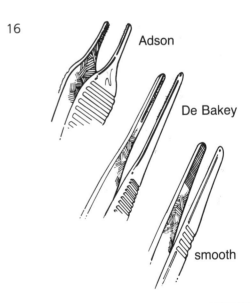

Adson

De Bakey

smooth

Forceps should be approximated with only the minimum pressure required to hold the tissue. Grasping can often be avoided by letting the inherent spring of the forceps hold the tissue apart for sewing or dissecting.

17a

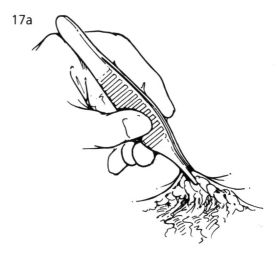

17b

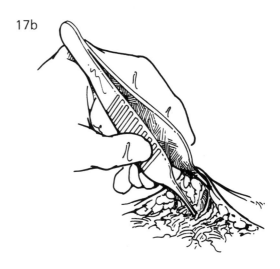

For right-handed operators, forceps are best held with the left hand. After prolonged use, forceps may lose their ability to grasp because the tips have separated or no longer are aligned. Mal-alignment can be readily seen by holding the forceps up to the light and can be remedied by placing a clamp near the tips to hold them apart and then, with the clamp as a lever, gently bending the tips back together with a second clamp.

TYING

The accompanying illustrations demonstrate the double-hand knot, the single-hand knot, and the instrument tie. Each of these has its advantages.

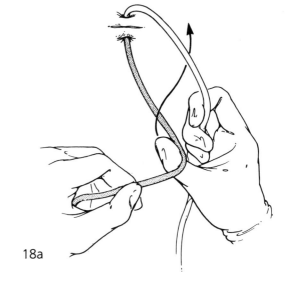

18a

Double-hand Knot

The double-hand knot is the most easily controlled of the three and is therefore used to ligate larger vessels and to approximate tissues with precision.

18b

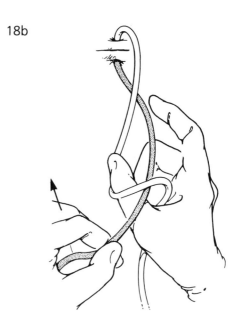

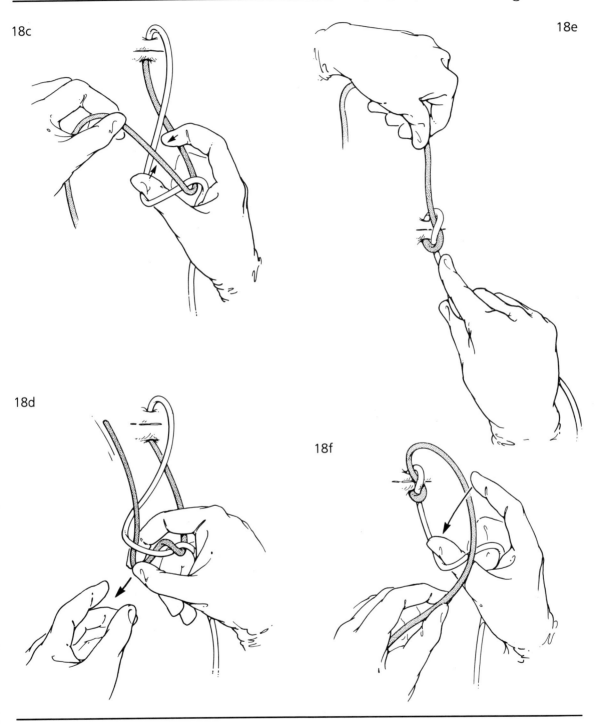

18c

18d

18e

18f

18g

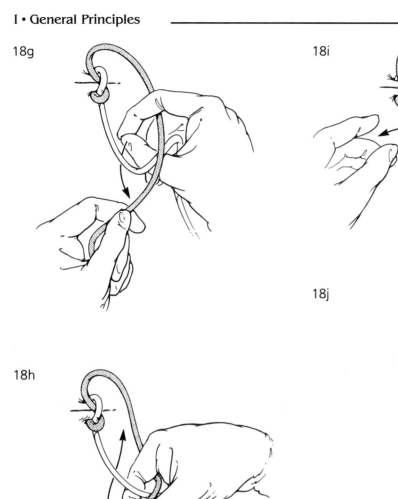

18i

18h

18j

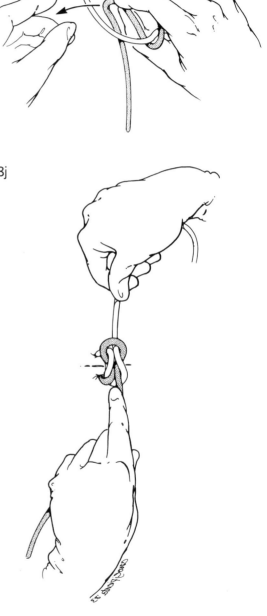

Single-hand Knot

The single-hand knot is fast and is therefore used when there are many sutures to be tied or in ligation of small vessels.

19a

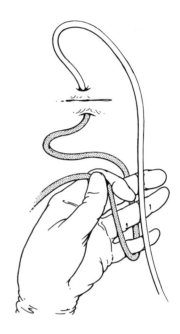

19b

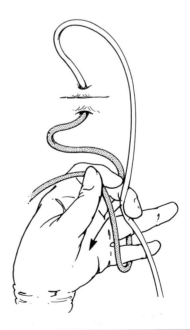

19c

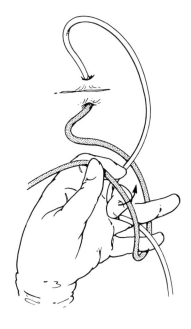

19e

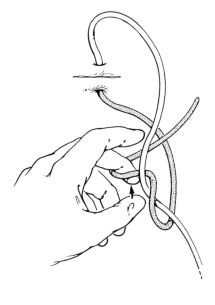

19d

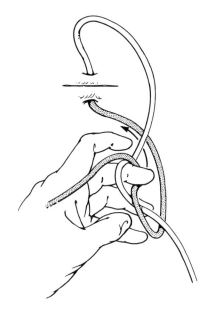

19f

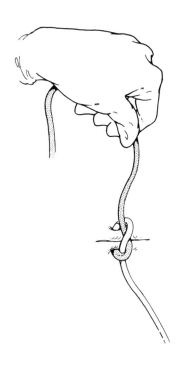

19g

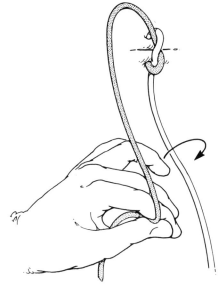

19i

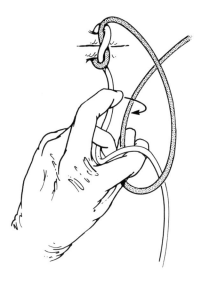

19h

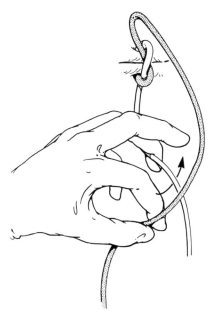

19j

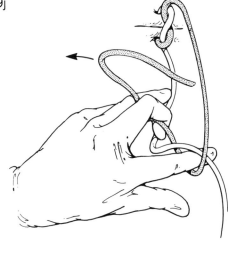

19k

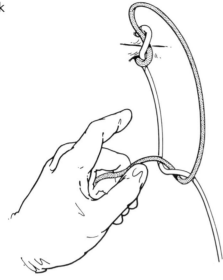

19l

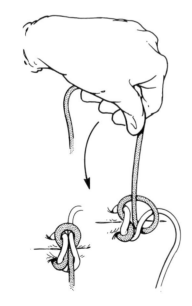

Instrument Tie

The instrument tie is also rapid and is particularly useful when there is a need to conserve the length of the suture—for example, in placement of multiple stitches during closure of a laceration.

20a

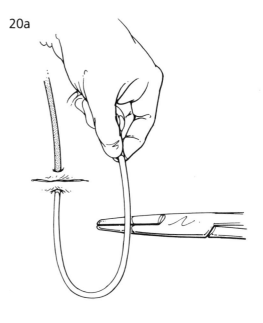

20b

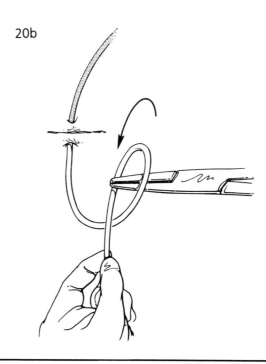

20c

20e

20d

20f

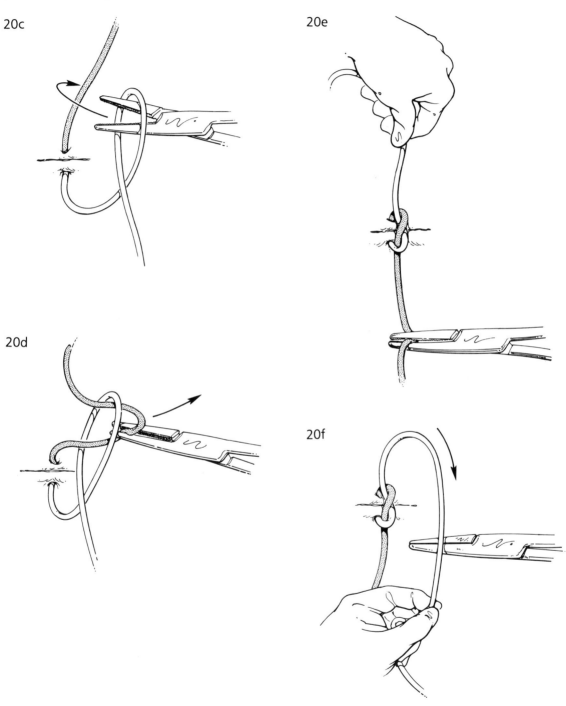

20g

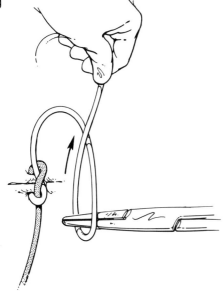

20i

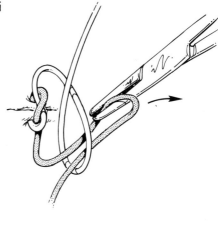

20h

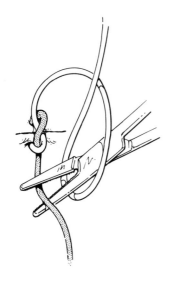

20j

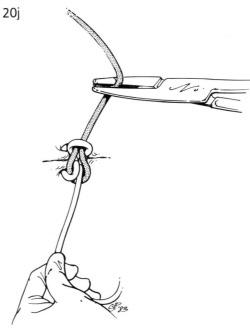

SEWING

The quality of the surgery is frequently judged by the neatness of the closure. This is not an inappropriate standard; a well-sewn wound heals well.

Sewing of the skin can be done rapidly and accurately with a hand-held needle such as the Keith straight cutting edge needle. The technique has two advantages: a minimum of equipment is required, and skin sutures can be placed with excellent precision.

21

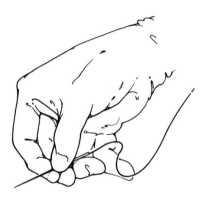

Needle holders are supplied in two designs, the common ratchet and the spring-loaded models. The ratchet holders are sturdier, easier to use, and considerably less expensive than the spring-loaded models.

Needle holders seem clumsy initially, but a little practice soon provides a feeling of confidence. The most important trick is to follow the curve of the needle with a smooth movement of the wrist; there should be no resistance during placement and follow-through of the needle. A bent or broken needle signals that the curve has not been followed. When the needle has been pushed through the tissues, it can be picked up with the forceps, but a better approach is to pick it up with a needle holder so that the next stitch can be placed without an additional motion.

In summary, even the most complex operations require only the basic manipulations of cutting, clamping, grasping, tying, and sewing. Each of these can be learned readily with relatively little practice, yielding great benefit to patients and to the office schedule. Specific approaches to the sewing of various wounds and tissues, the selection of stitches, and the choice of needles and suture materials are presented in Chapter 10.

5 · *Antisepsis and Draping of the Field*

FRANCIS T. THOMAS, M.D.

Antisepsis and draping of the field are important elements in office surgery because they minimize infection, demarcate and isolate the surgical area, protect the patient's clothing, and maintain the ambience compatible with a surgical procedure.

The patient should be comfortable during the procedure. Accordingly, he or she should empty the bladder, change to a gown, and assume the most comfortable position that is compatible with the planned operation.

Shaving is rarely needed. The nicks and abrasions produced by the shaving are more likely to cause infection than the hair. Particularly dangerous is the practice of shaving several hours prior to surgery; bacteria invade such a traumatized field widely and sharply increase the chance for a wound infection.

Shaving exposed areas such as the arms and head also produces an unsightly bald spot, which causes embarrassment by drawing attention to the operative site. Such a spot is ugly.

Even patients with a lesion under a luxuriant head of hair can be operated upon without shaving. The hair can be parted so that the part is in line with the proposed incision. If the area is then thoroughly washed with an antiseptic agent, the danger of infection is minimal, because the scalp has an excellent blood supply and great resistance to infection.

The choice of antiseptic agent is left to the surgeon. There are a number of excellent agents on the market. We prefer to use a combination of the povidone-iodine (Betadine) soap and Betadine solution. The combination is effective, well tolerated by most patients, and temporarily colors the treated area, thus clearly defining the boundaries of the prepared field. Betadine soap is useful for reducing bacteria to moderate levels but is not completely effective in reducing bacterial counts prior to surgical incision. Therefore, Betadine soap is first used to scrub the area to be operated upon. This will decrease the concentration of bacteria on the skin to levels of 10^2 to 10^3 per cubic centimeter and reduce the likelihood of infection considerably. Unless the lesion to be excised is a potentially malignant tumor such as a melanoma or other skin tumor that one would not want to manipulate excessively, a vigorous scrubbing with an iodine soap is in order. When a painful abscess is present, vigorous scrubbing is also unwise because of discomfort to the patient.

After the operative area has been scrubbed with the Betadine soap, it is dried and painted with the Betadine solution. The prep solution is much more bacteriostatic and bacteriocidal than the soap solution and can reduce the bacterial concentration by a factor of 10^6 or 10^7 organisms per cubic centimeter. In preparing the field, it is usually wise to wear and then discard a pair of sterile gloves, donning a new set for the operative procedure. Remember that Betadine solution discolors everything it touches, so be careful not to splash it on the patient's clothing. Also remember that Betadine or other iodophor agents should not be used to prepare patients who are allergic to iodine.

Many surgeons prefer preparation of the skin with a soap solution such as pHisoHex. This is a perfectly adequate skin prep, but studies have demonstrated that it does not reduce skin bacterial flora counts to the 10^4 level that one would like to see in most situations. It does call for rather vigorous scrubbing of the skin, and therefore it is not as easy or pleasant for the patient who is awake for office surgery as it is for the anesthetized patient in hospital surgery. This agent is effective against most gram-positive organisms, and it also provides much protection against many gram-negative bacteria. During an epidemic of *E. coli* wound infections at our institution, we were able to demonstrate the cause to be several pHisoHex dispensers that had been contaminated by and still sustained heavy colonization with these bacteria.

A solution of 70% denatured alcohol (ethyl alcohol solution) is one of the most bacteriostatic agents known, and there is little scientific evidence that any agent surpasses the capability of alcohol to reduce the numbers of bacteria on the skin. If the alcohol solution is colored with a preservative to give a slightly pink color, it will clearly delineate the area that has been prepared.

In my opinion, the Betadine soap-and-solution combination or a soap-and-alcohol combination is the preferred technique for antiseptic preparation of the skin. Again, it is important to note that areas such as the scalp, axilla, and the groin, pubic, and peritoneal areas require special attention to antisepsis.

Probably one of the best ways to prepare the skin is to ask the patient to bathe thoroughly and wash the hair with a deodorant antiseptic soap such as Lifebuoy or Irish Spring just before coming to the office. After the skin has been cleansed, the area of surgery is delineated with three or four sterile towels that are held together with towel clips. Care must be taken not to pinch the patient's skin as these are applied.

The physician may prefer to use disposable drapes that can be purchased with adhesive strips and precut holes, but we find these clumsy and expensive. It is hard to improve on the economy, efficiency, and adaptability of towels and towel clips.

If a break in surgical antisepsis occurs during the course of an operation, a regimen of antibiotics for a three-to-five-day period is indicated; also observe the patient carefully. Similarly, antibiotics may be indicated if the patient has an established infection, if the operation is done in a dirty area, if the patient is immunocompromised, or if the patient has had previous postoperative infections. An inexpensive cephalosporin such as Anspor or a broad-spectrum antibiotic such as tetracycline should be given in such instances. Antibiotics provide the best protection if they are administered before the incision is made; if an antibiotic is given after an operation because a break in technique has occurred, it should be given promptly and in high dosage to effect a high blood level as quickly as possible.

The practitioner who does not use prophylactic antibiotics may find him- or herself subject to criticism from patients and others despite the fact that prophylactic antibiotics are probably overused. In a similar vein, a physician being sued in a case of infection will be hard put to defend his or her decision not to administer antibiotics in a questionable situation. The general rule ought to be no antibiotics in clean cases, prophylactic antibiotics in doubtful cases, and antibiotics in infected cases.

In summary, antisepsis and preparation of the field for operation are critical steps in outpatient surgery. The potential for a break in antiseptic technique is far greater than in hospital surgery. Prophylactic antibiotics should be given for a short time whenever there is a possibility of infection due to a break in sterile technique or in an immunocompromised patient.

6 · *Anesthesia for Office Surgery*

WALTER J. PORIES, M.D.

Anesthesia for office surgery is local anesthesia. Although the new ambulatory surgical centers attest to the safety of general, spinal, and regional anesthesia for outpatient surgery, these techniques are rarely used in the office of the family physician because they require specialized equipment and sophisticated monitoring and may be associated with serious complications.

Reassurance and appropriate preparation are important initial steps in successful local anesthesia. The procedure and its various steps need to be explained to the patient and often to the accompanying companion, guardian, or parent. If the patient seems unduly anxious, about either the procedure or the implications of the biopsy, sedation with medications given orally, such as sodium pentobarbital (100 mg) or diazepam (5 mg), can be a great help. Sedation may also be given during the procedure by the IV route; we find 1 to 2 mg of diazepam, administered slowly, to be an effective agent.

The patient needs to be in a comfortable position and not so swathed in drapes that he or she becomes claustrophobic or anxious about obtaining enough air. It is helpful to keep talking to the patient during the procedure to reassure that the operation is progressing satisfactorily. One of the important tasks of the nurse circulating in the room is to soothe and comfort, as well as to monitor, the patient.

Commonly Used Solutions of Lidocaine

Concentration, %	Administration	Application
0.5	Intradermal, subcutaneous	Local anesthesia for large volumes of tissue, multiple locations
1	Intradermal, subcutaneous, perineural	Most uses, local and regional anesthesia, nerve blocks
2	Mucosal, perineural	Topical anesthesia, nerve blocks
4	Mucosal, perineural	Topical anesthesia, nerve blocks

Lidocaine, the most widely used agent for local anesthesia, is available in various concentrations, as shown in the table above.

Whatever concentration is used, the dosage of lidocaine should not exceed 500 mg—for example, 50 ml of a 1% solution, 25 ml of a 2% solution, or 12.5 ml of a 4% solution. Beyond these dosages, toxic symptoms are not uncommon. Accordingly, care must be used not to exceed these volumes in patients with multiple lacerations or who require anesthesia in large volumes of tissue. If adequate anesthesia cannot be obtained within these guidelines, it is safer to consider other approaches such as general anesthesia or regional block; these alternatives may require more sophisticated facilities such as a hospital or a free-standing ambulatory surgical center. In those isolated, remote, and rare situations where no other answer except local anesthesia is feasible and the repair cannot be completed rapidly, the procedure may be staged to allow metabolism of the anesthetic, with the two stages of the repair separated by 3 to 4 hr.

The toxic symptoms of overdosage usually appear insidiously but may progress rather rapidly to dangerous manifestations. The earliest signs include anxiety, garrulousness, and agitation; if these are not recognized and the overdosage corrected, and especially if additional lidocaine is given, the picture may quickly progress to arrhythmias, confusion, seizures, and even death. If a patient becomes agitated and excessively talkative during a procedure under lidocaine anesthesia, do not inject any more of the anesthetic, and begin an IV solution, sedate the patient with barbiturate or diazepam, and finish the procedure expeditiously.

Local anesthetics such as lidocaine can also cause allergic reactions and anaphylactic shock. *Always inquire carefully regarding allergies to procaine hydrochloride (Novocain), lidocaine, and other local anesthetic agents before administering lidocaine.* I once caused a cardiac arrest in a physician by injecting only a drop or two of lidocaine, at most, under his skin in preparation for the excision of a small mole. Fortunately, resuscitation was fully successful. Therefore, the following rules are important:

• Always ask regarding allergies and any previous experience with the drug to be used.

• Never do office surgery without someone else in the room.

• Be certain that the drugs and equipment needed for surgical emergencies are immediately available.

Epinephrine added to the lidocaine minimizes capillary ooze and prolongs the action of the local anesthesia by slowing diffusion, absorption, and metabolism of the agent through local vasoconstriction. This vasoconstrictive effect is useful in most cases, but epinephrine represents a hazard to patients with high blood pressure, heart disease, and arrhythmias and should be used in such patients with caution. Epinephrine is also a hazard when it is injected into tissues with limited circulation. Do not use it in areas such as the nose, ears, fingers, toes, and penis. Even a small area of gangrene in any of these areas is a major complication; the loss of the glans penis, a finger, or the tip of the nose is a catastrophe. In short, if there is a question about the effect of epinephrine, don't use it.

A particularly dangerous practice is the use of rubber bands as tourniquets on fingers or on the penis. Although the effectiveness of the local anesthetic can be prolonged by this technique, there have been too many instances where the rubber band was forgotten or not removed and the digit or organ was lost through ischemic gangrene. Accordingly, do not use a rubber band, rubber drain, or other device either to prolong anesthesia or to control bleeding.

Following are some helpful hints for making local anesthesia as comfortable as possible:

1. Ask yourself whether local anesthesia is even needed. Aspiration of lesions such as breast cysts can be done comfortably without anesthesia if the skin is punctured quickly and only once with a sharp needle, even as large as a #18. If a larger needle is needed, an anesthetic is probably advisable. Repairs of small lacerations can often be made with adhesive strips or with one or two quick closures with one of the new disposable skin-stapling devices.

2. For economy, use the lidocaine in the 50-ml vial. Be certain to use a new needle and syringe at each aspiration to avoid contamination of the bottle. Withdrawal of the anesthetic is best done through a large needle, either a #18 or #20, and not through the #25 used for injection; the aspiration is easier through the larger bore, and the fine needle may lose its point when it is pushed through the rubber cap.

3. Use a #25 or #26 needle to inject the anesthetic. Minimize the number of injections by using a long needle. If several skin punctures are needed, use more than one needle to assure that you always have a sharp point.

4. If an incision is to be made, mark the site with an indelible pen to guide the injec-

tion of the anesthetic. A properly administered local anesthetic will not leave visible evidence; the dotted line assures that the incision will be made in the anesthetized area. The marker also serves to remind you to administer additional anesthetic if you need to extend your incision or extension.

5. Inject the anesthetic slowly, almost imperceptibly. Rapid injection is painful. Make the initial wheal by injecting only a drop of the lidocaine just under the skin. Wait 30 to 40 sec, then *very slowly* inject the anesthetic throughout the required area, placing most of it under the skin. When the anesthetic has been injected, massage the area gently for 2 to 3 min before proceeding.

6. To avoid an intravascular administration, draw the plunger back briefly before injecting the anesthetic to make sure there is no backflow of blood.

7. Save the injured patient considerable pain by injecting the lidocaine through the edges of the wound rather than the intact skin and anesthetizing lacerations before the area is scrubbed and cleansed. Repair of lacerations can be made almost totally painless by first dripping a milliliter or so of 1% lidocaine into the wound and waiting several minutes for absorption of the agent by the exposed tissues. The additional anesthetic is then injected slowly under the surrounding skin and into the depths of the wound *through* the injured tissues. The laceration can then be scrubbed and debrided with minimal discomfort.

8. If the procedure is expected to involve deeper tissues, such as in a lymph node or muscle biopsy, be prepared to inject additional anesthetic during the course of the operation. Frequently question the patient about discomfort. When the patient complains or shows other signs of pain, stop operating and slowly infiltrate more lidocaine.

9. Arteries are unusually sensitive and somewhat resistant to the local anesthetic. If an artery 1 mm or larger requires clamping or a ligature, inject its wall with a drop or two of lidocaine before proceeding.

10. Keep careful records of the type and amount of anesthetic used.

11. Observe the patient for an hour or more to be certain that there are no untoward reactions such as a rash, hemorrhage, anaphylaxis, or failure of neurologic function, motor or sensory, to return.

The nerve block is a useful approach for the induction of local anesthesia in selected anatomic areas such as the fingers, toes, penis, anus, and regions of the face. Nerve blocks are usually performed with 2% or 4% lidocaine anesthesia injected about the perineurium in small amounts—0.5 to 1 ml at each site.

Nerve blocks of the fingers and toes can be achieved fairly easily with minimal discomfort. The needle is pushed through the skin to the bone at each side of the digit, and about 0.5 ml of lidocaine is injected. The needle is then withdrawn and redirected 45 degrees superiorly and inferiorly to the neurovascular bundle, as shown in Chapter 25, on each side. This should achieve good anesthesia of the digit; if the anesthesia is not complete, a ring of anesthetic solution can be injected around the base of the digit to assure total insensitivity.

The technique for inducing a nerve block of the penis is shown in Chapter 22.

7 · Biopsies and Excision of Lesions

WALTER J. PORIES, M.D.

Biopsies and excisions of lesions are not diffi-cult. If the family physician is prepared to do these procedures, the patient is saved a referral, delay, and, often, considerable cost. If further treatment is called for, the patient can still be referred to the appropriate specialist, with the advantage that the problem has already been identified.

The stage should be set before the patient en-ters the operating room. The operative consent should have been signed, the procedure should have been fully explained, and the antiseptic and anesthetic agents, surgical instruments, su-tures, and dressings should be prepared and in

their place. Of particular importance is the read-iness of a fully equipped crash cart for prompt, effective handling of the rare but possible event of anaphylactic shock, cardiac arrest, drug re-action, or other complications.

SKIN LESIONS

Shaving is rarely needed in excising skin lesions. We have noted no increased incidence of in-fection since we have stopped shaving patients; the patients are grateful that they do not have to explain a bald spot or endure the itch of regrowing hair.

The operative area is gently washed with Betadine soap. Other organic povidone-iodine preparations and in fact other antiseptics are probably equally satisfactory, but we continue to use Betadine because it is well tolerated, appears to provide effective protection, and temporarily colors the operative area to show the extent of the skin preparation. Another advantage of Betadine is that it can be easily washed off the skin after the operation. Many surgeons prep the skin with a sponge stick (a folded 4-×4-in sponge held in a ring forceps); we prefer to use our hands to hold the antiseptic-soaked sponge, a more effective, less clumsy, and gentler method.

1

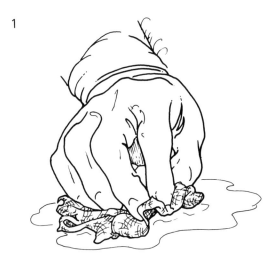

Wounds heal far better if they are made in the direction of wrinkle lines. If possible, excision lines should follow these natural guides; the final scars are far less noticeable if this rule is followed. Even a wound that has to be opened because of infection will heal into a fine scar if it was made within the wrinkle lines. Wrinkle lines can be found throughout the body and are readily demonstrated by gentle pinching of the skin, as shown in Figure 4, Chapter 4. Hair can also serve as a guide; it usually (but not always) grows in the direction of the wrinkle lines.

2

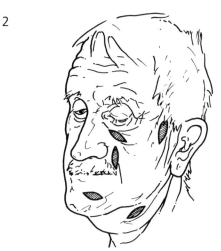

The area to be excised, with a margin of at least 1 cm (in three dimensions) is liberally infiltrated with 1% lidocaine; the injection should be done slowly with a very fine (#25) needle. The injection, painful if too rapid, can be totally painless if done very slowly—namely, 1 ml in the first minute. Additional amounts can be injected more quickly as the anesthesia develops.

3

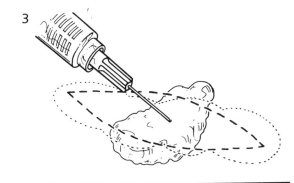

The addition of epinephrine cuts bleeding sharply. We use it universally *except in the fingers, toes, nose, ears, nipples, and penis* because in each of these areas there is danger of gangrene from ischemia. Epinephrine does make some patients anxious because of its side effects; we therefore may also omit this agent in patients who are unduly nervous about the procedure.

Delineation of the proposed incision with a ballpoint pen is often useful. Although the ink is often washed away during the prep, a fine red welt caused by dermographia will usually remain to guide the cuts. A fine-point Magic Marker with permanent ink can also be used but often leaves a dark line that may be hard to remove.

4

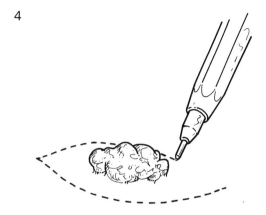

Most skin lesions, such as nevi, warts, or papillomata, require only a 1- to 2-cm margin on all sides *and deep to* the lesion. The incisions are extended in the direction of the wrinkle lines to give a boat shape to the specimen, so that a smooth closure can be effected.

5

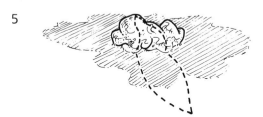

If the lesion is too large for excision, the incisional biopsy should include a strip of tissue representing the most abnormal part of the lesion and extending back to normal skin.

The excision of sebaceous cysts or infected sinuses should always include the pore or cutaneous opening.

6

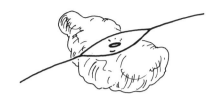

The excision of lymph nodes that are deep to the skin need not include a piece of the overlying skin.

7

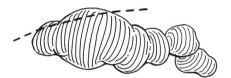

The excision is best done with a #15 scalpel, held like a pen. The tissue is tightened with traction by the other hand to keep the field stable, allow clean cuts, and minimize bleeding. With constant traction, which admittedly does take some practice, it is often possible to remove a skin lesion with a totally dry field and no blood loss whatever.

8

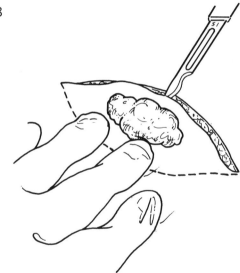

Traction (and, with it, the control of bleeding) is maintained during the deep part of the excision by clamping and pulling on the edge of the specimen.

9

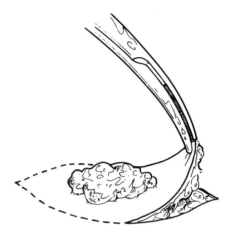

Several small bleeders are usually present in the base and on the edges of the wound. These can usually be controlled with a gentle touch of the cautery. Larger bleeders may need to be clamped for more effective cauterization or may even require ligature with a 4-0 absorbable suture such as Vicryl or Dexon.

10

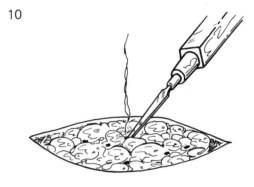

Most small excision sites can be closed with a subcuticular suture of 4-0 Vicryl (see Chapter 10), but if there is any tension, a closure with continuous or interrupted skin stitches of 4-0 or 5-0 Prolene is preferable.

11

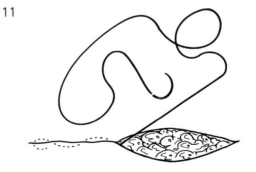

NODE BIOPSIES

Node biopsies are more difficult than excision of skin lesions. Lymph nodes are often deeper than they seem to be on palpation, the tissue is more friable, and there is often a profuse blood supply.

Usually a layer of muscle, such as platysma, or a layer of fascia, such as Scarpa's, must be divided to expose the node. A small self-retaining retractor is useful in improving exposure and minimizing bleeding by traction.

12

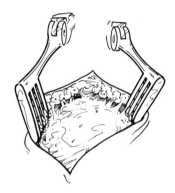

The node is freed by gently pushing other tissues away from its capsule. Vessels should be clamped and cauterized as they are exposed; they may be difficult to control if allowed to retract into the depth of the wound.

13

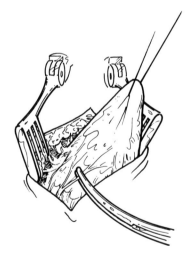

The main node is usually attached to several other nodes, and these can often be removed to yield additional material for examination or culture.

14

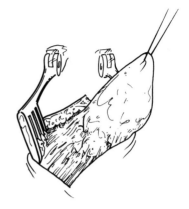

If a node is too large to be removed, a wedge of the tissues can be taken in biopsy.

15

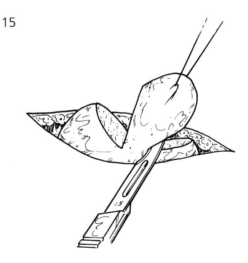

Whether the node is excised or taken in biopsy by excision of a wedge, the specimen should be protected from crushing by holding it with a suture or not holding it at all until it is fully freed.

It is too easy to lose the specimen in the drapes and during the cleanup. As soon as the specimen has been excised, it should be handed to the assistant, placed immediately in the appropriate specimen container, and labeled. Notations about orientation of the specimen are often helpful to the pathologist.

16

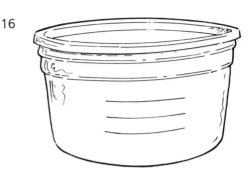

The node should be divided into several pieces. The largest should be saved for the pathologist, and several smaller pieces should be sent for the culture of acid-fast bacilli and fungal and other bacterial organisms.

17

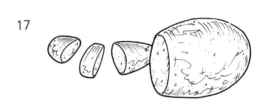

A half-inch Steri-strip is an almost ideal dressing; it splints the skin for better healing, serves to cushion the wound, makes the wound less sensitive to touch, and is cosmetically acceptable. If a layer of tincture of benzoin is applied before application of the Steri-strip, it will stick well enough to allow the patient to bathe without disturbing it.

18

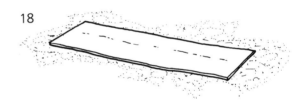

Patients should be cautioned to be careful of any site of excision and to protect it from injury, soiling, and overuse. Aspirin, Darvocet, or codeine will usually minimize discomfort; if these analgesics do not control the pain, or if there are indications of local or systemic infection, the patient should be seen promptly to determine whether there is a complication. The sutures can usually be removed after one week except when the excision site is in an extremity, in which case two weeks may be needed for healing. Healing is also slower in the elderly and in patients with systemic disease. If in doubt, leave the sutures in a few more days.

8 · *Preparing and Handling the Specimen*

FRANCIS T. THOMAS, M.D.

In the course of office surgery, the practitioner may obtain a variety of specimens: for example, fluid requiring chemical analysis or cell analysis, aspirates obtained by aspiration biopsy with a fine needle, tissue cores obtained by needle biopsy, and solid tissue specimens obtained by incisional or excisional biopsy.

Analysis of any of these specimens may be performed in the office using simple techniques (usually a Gram's stain or other microbacterial analysis) or in a pathology lab (either free standing or associated with a medical facility). Laboratory analysis of such specimens may be an extremely valuable aid to diagnosis, and it calls for close cooperation between pathologist and surgeon. The pathologist should be given in-

formation about the clinical history and other pertinent data to help in the clarification of the histopathological or microbiological diagnosis. The surgeon should always indicate clearly to the pathologist or laboratory analyst precisely what he or she is looking for, giving details of the clinical history and findings. The specimen must be taken and handled properly. Labeling must be precise. The report from the pathologist must be returned promptly, and there must be a mechanism in the office for early review of the report and notification of the patient.

The pathologic diagnosis is by its nature incomplete because it represents a single laboratory examination. Often, too, the cellular or microbiological nature of the specimen may belie the clinical course and prognosis of the disease process. With more modern techniques (e.g., monoclonal antibody studies of tumor cell markers) the pathologist may be able to predict the nature, course, and prognosis of a disease more accurately than the clinician who is relying on the history or physical examination. The best communication between clinician and pathologist calls for free interaction and discussion of a particular case. Many pathologists like both to be consulted before or at the time of a biopsy and to discuss directly with the clinician interpretation of the biopsy. Both pathologist and surgeon must be certain they are using the same terminology. Many medical terms are interpreted loosely and often in a contradictory manner by different specialists.

Obtaining specimens, analyzing them, accurately reporting results, and interpreting them make up a complex process with many medicolegal overtones. Areas in which pathologist and surgeon are most vulnerable to litigation include labeling and handling of specimens, interpretation, prompt transmittal of interpretation to the surgeon, further transmittal to the patient, and careful follow-up to ensure that the diagnosis is followed by the appropriate therapy. Because the surgical practitioner and the pathologist are often geographically separated, there is potential for serious errors of communication.

For several centuries, practitioners have examined specimens containing microorganisms. Until this century, microorganism infections were the leading cause of death in most countries. Even today, microorganisms are a large cause of morbidity and mortality and, despite improved public health measures, continue to plague humankind. Recently, the advent of immunosuppression and chemotherapy has produced unusual pathology caused by microorganisms having no previous association with active disease, making accurate analysis of bacteriological specimens very important to patient care.

Several types of specimens may be examined for microbacteria, but the specimen so analyzed is usually fluid, often pus. Fluid infected with large concentrations of bacteria often is odoriferous and turbid; a practitioner can often make a preliminary diagnosis by the appearance and smell of the material. When pus is obtained by aspiration or biopsy in the office, immediate examination of the fluid with a microscope and the familiar Gram's stain is usually helpful. It is good practice to have such materials at hand to determine whether the predominant organisms are gram-negative or gram-positive and to identify typical forms such as rods or the familiar cluster of staphylococcal infection. Guided by the Gram's stain preparation, even before culture and sensitivity tests are carried out, reasonably accurate antibiotic therapy can be started since the morphology of the organism and its positive- or negative-staining characteristics often give strong clues as to the appropriate antibiotic to use.

For the Gram's stain, make a light smear of pus across a slide, add the Gram's stain, and dry the slide. After washing, the slide is ready to be examined. In making smears, take bacteriologic precautions; the nature of the infection is not known, and the organisms may be highly contagious. When acid-fast organisms are suspected, it is especially important to ensure that the organisms and specimen are properly disposed of. Smears may also be obtained from solid tissue, such as a lymph node, by scraping or impression.

Cultures, formerly smeared directly onto agar plates, are now almost always inoculated into commercially available plastic tubes, with an attached sterile cotton-tip applicator. Material to be cultured can also be placed in commercially available trypsin soy broth (Bactec, Johnson Laboratories, Towson, MD).

For anaerobic bacteria, kits are now commercially available with an inner flask containing a chemical that, when the flask is broken, acts to remove oxygen from the culture tube. Anaerobic organisms, a very large cause of significant morbidity and mortality in human disease, must be identified. Such organisms will not grow unless anaerobic conditions are provided; thus, the anaerobic culture tube is essential. The Bactec anaerobic trypsin soy broth is also very effective in selecting for anaerobes.

Send specimens for culture to the pathology laboratory as soon as possible. If your office is distant from the laboratory and facilities are not available for immediate transport, the specimen may be stored for a period usually not to exceed 24 hr, provided storage is under adequate refrigeration, both for bacteriologic specimens and for tissue specimens fixed in formalin.

An unfortunate mistake often made in obtaining bacteriological specimens or other tissue is incorrect labeling, usually the result of failure to affix immediately a label with the patient's name and patient identification number when the specimen is obtained. The label must be sealed securely to the specimen container, not merely wrapped around it or placed in a box or bag with it. An accompanying specimen form should state clearly the patient's name and identifying number, the date the specimen was obtained, provenance of the specimen, the considered diagnosis or differential diagnoses, and a brief clinical history.

In filling out the pathology form, provide adequate data to help the pathologist, including the potential disease process and what you suspect the specimen might show. Remember that a given specimen may be examined by many different methods. For example, a pleural effusion can be examined to determine whether it is an exudate, and whether it contains a high or low percentage of leucocytes, a high or low percentage of lymphocytes, free-floating tumor cells, amylase in high concentrations, and many other characterizations, all of which may help greatly in establishing the diagnosis.

Biopsy specimens may be obtained by fine-needle aspiration or by incisional or excisional biopsy. Fine-needle aspiration is a valuable technique, which has become popular recently. The method allows taking an adequate biopsy specimen through a very fine needle, minimizing morbidity from the procedure. For larger specimens, the Tru/cut needle biopsy technique has been steadily rising in popularity since the commercial introduction of such needles. The disposable needles are always sharp and functional, and, because they are intended for single use, any contamination by pathological material is disposed of along with the needle. The technique is well illustrated on the package insert accompanying the needle. The outer needle is placed over the inner core needle and then passed into the tissue to be sampled, cutting out a core of tissue, which is then withdrawn from the field and deposited in a container. This small core of tissue can be lost easily in the process of dislodging it; care should be taken to avoid such an event.

Specimens removed by biopsy should be placed in 10% formalin with a neutral buffer, a solution which can maintain tissue in optimal condition for examination for a period of months to years. The volume of formalin should be at least ten times as large as the volume of tissue.

In my surgery practice, all such tissues are placed in plastic containers; we no longer use glass containers because they break if dropped.

Sophisticated techniques are indicated for analyzing lymph nodes, since a wide variety of lymphatic tumors are now recognized, each with a differing prognosis; also, some benign diseases such as infectious mononucleosis can resemble aggressive lymphatic tumors. Monoclonal antibody testing can identify T and B cell markers and can indicate whether tumor cells in a lymph node are so-called polyclonal or monoclonal. Monoclonal lymph node cells are almost inevitably tumors, whereas polyclonal cells often indicate an inflammatory response. A new patient with an unknown diagnosis and large groups of lymph nodes carries a heavy suspicion of cancer. In such a case, an entire lymph node should be removed as soon as possible so that at least 1 gm (1 cc) of tissue is obtained. A portion of this should be frozen as soon as possible. The surgeon should place the fresh lymph node in a solution such as Michel's solution, which renders the tissue satisfactory for immunofluorescence and immunoperoxidase or other immunochemical studies with markers. A portion of the lymph node should also be placed in the standard 10% formalin solution for routine chemical examination. The tissue should then be transported as soon as possible to the pathologist.

For pathological specimens including lymphomas of the skin or any potential skin tumor, sutures or other markers may be helpful to the pathologist for orientation. One should resist the temptation to slice a specimen open while it is fresh; doing so often produces an uneven specimen after formalin fixation. If the specimen is greater than 3 cm in any dimension or if there is likely to be a delay of two or more days before the specimen reaches the pathol-

ogist, the specimen should be cut up into smaller pieces to permit more adequate penetration of the tissue by the formalin, orientation indicators being preserved, and the tissue should be refrigerated if more than 24 hr will elapse from time of excision to transport to the pathology lab.

The Papanicolaou, or Pap, smear used to detect cervical carcinoma or precancerous lesions has greatly reduced the morbidity and mortality attendant upon cervical carcinoma, which is entirely curable in its early stages. Most people feel that all women over the age of 30 should have a yearly Pap smear. This is a simple test with simple techniques. Pap smears are easily obtained during the course of a pelvic examination, following insertion of a vaginal speculum, with the patient in the lithotomy position. The cervix is visualized and cleared of any gross mucus. The special curved, wooden, Pap smear stick is swept around all four quadrants of the cervix to obtain a specimen. If such a stick is not available, a tongue blade will serve. The vaginal speculum can be used to rotate the cervix to a position affording greater ease of scraping. These scrapings are then placed on a glass slide, fixed in absolute alcohol, and sent to the pathology lab. A cotton-tip applicator is then inserted into the cervical os so as to obtain specimens from both the cervical epithelium and the columnar-squamous junction. This smear is placed on a separate slide. The two slides should be labeled "endocervix" and "ectocervix." The second slide is also fixed in alcohol and sent to the pathology lab for examination. Make sure that the endocervical specimen is ample; cancer cannot be ruled out unless both squamous and columnar epithelia are present to show that the smear is completely representative of the columnar-squamous junction.

There are hundreds of tests for identification of

unusual microorganisms and unusual types of solid lesions, including immunofluorescence studies, antigen studies for microorganisms, antibody studies, immunoperoxidase studies, complement-fixation studies, and electron microscopy of solid lesions. The practical value of some such tests has not been established. After obtaining a specimen, it is wise to consult with a pathologist who has expert knowledge in these areas. The tests are often expensive; since the diagnoses are often rare and many of the ailments can only be treated symptomatically, one must think of the cost-effectiveness of such tests, particularly in the case of viral diseases, such as herpes, which can be treated only symptomatically.

The immunocompromised patient requires very careful medical management. Such patients can develop many infections, both common and unusual, and specimens obtained from these people require careful study. Sometimes the called-for tests are esoteric ones that can only be performed by specialized state laboratories or the excellent facilities at the Centers for Disease Control in Atlanta, Georgia. A practitioner would be wise to seek expert advice regarding appropriate laboratory studies and treatment for the immunocompromised patient.

9 · Management of the Traumatic Wound: Debridement

WALTER J. PORIES, M.D.

Although management of seriously traumatized wounds is not a problem normally encountered by the family physician, it is included here because the principles involved are relevant to all wound care and because any physician might find him- or herself caring for major wounds—for example, in wartime, at the scene of accidents, in the emergency room, in a rural practice, and during disasters.

The first concern in the care of traumatic wounds is the overall condition of the patient. The well-known ABCs of resuscitation—airway, breathing, and circulation—must be addressed first. Only when the patient's condition is reasonably stable should the wound be treated, especially if considerable additional bleeding is expected

during the debridement. It is particularly important to restore the patient's blood volume; hypovolemic patients tolerate even minimal surgery poorly. The patient should also be given tetanus toxoid and protected with prophylactic broad-spectrum antibiotics.

Initial care of the traumatic injury includes control of hemorrhage, shielding of exposed tissues from the environment, and splintage. Bleeding can almost always be controlled by pressure. In general, the pressure is more effective if it is exerted with a minimum number of sponges placed as precisely as possible at the bleeding site. Large, bulky dressings usually do not work because they do not permit effective pressure and can soak up an enormous amount of blood.

Similarly, reinforcement of dressings is often dangerous because it merely hides the continuing loss of blood, concealing from the physician the need for a more vigorous approach.

In those unusual instances where pressure does not arrest the bleeding, a tourniquet may be needed during transport, but it must be released at the earliest opportunity. Too many limbs and lives have been lost from unwise use of tourniquets. The ideal approach to hemorrhage is precise clamping of the bleeding vessels, but this method must be deferred until the patient's condition has become stable and until adequate help, light, and instruments are available. Hemostatic pressure can, at times, also be exerted with the MAST trousers or inflatable splints. These measures can control venous bleeding but are usually ineffective against arterial hemorrhage.

The cause of injury usually determines the amount of tissue damage to be found in a wound. Cuts made by knives or other sharp instruments usually produce the least tissue damage; high velocity missiles cause the most.

1a

The degree of cutaneous injury is not always a reliable indicator; high-velocity bullets, such as those from an M-16 rifle, frequently produce a wound of entry only 5 to 6 mm in diameter that hides an extensive area of tissue destruction measuring 20 to 30 cm. Similarly, crushing injuries, electrical burns, blunt trauma, and avulsions often produce extensive hidden areas of tissue destruction. A high degree of suspicion is a helpful rule.

1b

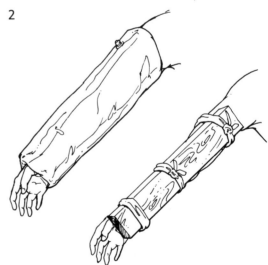

Splintage is an important adjunct to good wound care. It minimizes further damage from sharp bone spicules and helps prevent further bleeding and additional contamination from grinding of foreign materials within the wound. Finally, it controls pain and thus circumvents the likelihood of shock. Splints are usually readily available, but when they are not, they can easily be improvised from a variety of materials such as folded newspapers, branches, or pieces of lumber. The see-through plastic inflatable splints are particularly excellent because they are readily stored, are easy to apply, and provide hemostatic pressure.

2

DEBRIDEMENT AND MANAGEMENT OF INJURED TISSUES

All traumatic wounds are potentially infected with aerobic and anaerobic organisms. Although prophylactic antibiotics are indicated, they cannot be relied upon to protect the patient from infection. Only debridement—removal of dead and damaged tissues and diligent cleansing of foreign materials—will accomplish this end. The importance of debridement cannot be overstressed; if it is not done thoroughly and if the wound is not absolutely clean, tetanus, gas gangrene, and an extending, necrotizing, and advancing fasciitis may rapidly involve the wound, necessitating emergency amputation or causing the death of the patient.

Skin

The first step in debridement is the development of exposure by extending the wound with an incision in the direction of the wrinkle lines. Good debridement requires excellent exposure; every nook and cranny of the wound must be visible so that areas of damage and foreign bodies are not overlooked.

3

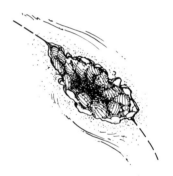

The skin is usually well supplied with blood vessels and considerably resistant to infection. Accordingly, debridement of skin is conservative; usually only a narrow edge of the skin needs to be sacrificed from the edges of the wound. Purple, discolored, crushed, and macerated skin should be excised; if there is a questionable area, it can be saved for later inspection. Scissors do this task much better than a scalpel.

4

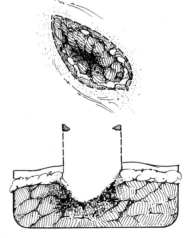

Muscle

In contrast to skin, muscle must be debrided and sacrificed radically. Any discolored, bruised, or noncontractile muscle must be totally excised, and all pockets must be laid open so that the wound is saucerized and able to drain freely. All nonmetallic foreign materials must be removed, especially bits of earth, projectile wads, or clothing; deeply buried and covered metallic objects such as bullets or shell fragments may be left in place if the removal requires too much additional time or tissue destruction. Debridement of muscle is best done with a forceps and scalpel or scissors and should be continued until all surfaces have the appearance of clean, red flesh. Often a jet of saline solution from a suspended IV bottle or a commercial apparatus such as the Waterpik will help to remove much of the loose material.

5

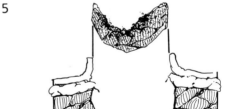

Bone

Bone should be saved if possible. All *detached* fragments should be removed and set aside under sterile conditions in an antibiotic solution (1 million units of penicillin and 1 gm of kanamycin or a similar solution) and refrigerated for possible use in later reconstruction as a bone graft. All *attached* fragments are gently cleaned with a curette or a rongeur and replaced in their normal positions when possible. The wound is then thoroughly lavaged with copious amounts of saline.

6

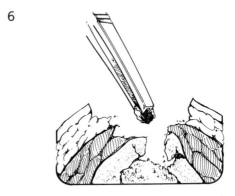

Although the bone occasionally can be left exposed, a preferable approach is to cover it with soft tissue by approximating nearby muscle over it with several lightly tied absorbable sutures. Internal fixation—the use of rods, nails, or plates—is not normally attempted if the wound is likely to become infected.

7

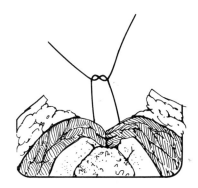

Joints

Joints have little resistance to infection and are rapidly destroyed by it. If a joint capsule is open in the base of a wound, it must be cleansed thoroughly. Remove the bone fragments and liberally irrigate the joint with saline and an antibiotic (0.5 gm kanamycin or Neosporin in 500 ml of saline). The edges of the capsule are approximated with fine sutures of an absorbable material such as Vicryl or Dexon. If possible, the capsule is then covered with viable soft tissue such as muscle or skin. No drain is used.

8

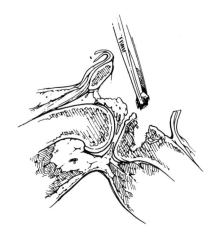

9

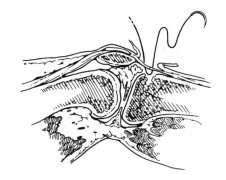

The wounded limb is immobilized by a thickly padded plaster cast. In major traumatic injuries it is important to bivalve the cast all the way down to the skin in anticipation of inevitable swelling of the extremity; if the cast is not split, there is a high risk of ischemia, Volkmann's contracture, or both. The fingers or toes must be checked frequently during the first 24 hr for capillary return, warmth, motion, and sensation. If there is any question about these indicators, or if the patient appears to have excessive pain, the cast should be changed.

10

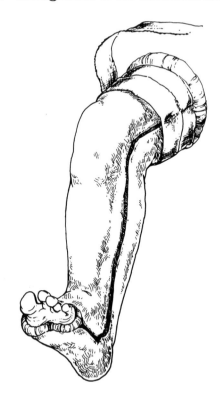

Tendons and Fascia

Both tendons and fascia have little resistance to infection because of their poor blood supply. These tissues must therefore be debrided widely, and if they are frayed, badly contaminated, or discolored, they should be removed.

Blood Vessels

The repair of blood vessels is difficult and is only included here for completeness. Arterial injuries are frequently more extensive than they appear at the initial examination. The circulation of the extremity should be checked frequently; pallor, pain, and pulselessness are late signs of vascular compromise. If there is any question of vascular injury or if the wound is near a major vessel, the patient should be moved to a facility where an arteriogram can be done without delay.

The principles of arterial repair include proximal and distal control by gently applied tapes or specially designed vascular clamps. Damaged vascular tissue is excised because it cannot be repaired well and the incidence of postrepair thrombosis is high. Arteries are repaired, if possible, by careful end-to-end approximation with a fine nonabsorbable suture such as 5-0 or 6-0 Prolene. If this is not feasible, the gap is bridged with a vein graft, usually from the saphenous vein. Whatever the approach, the repair must *not* be made under tension. Vascular prostheses, such as Dacron or Gortex, are not used in areas where they are likely to become infected; if there is no other alternative, these grafts can be routed extra-anatomically—that is, through areas not involved in the injury.

11

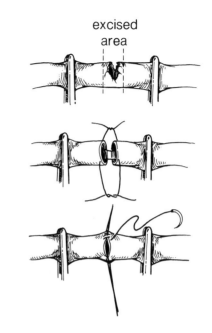

excised
area

Small veins can be ligated, but large veins, especially in distal extremities, should be repaired in the same fashion as arteries. Venous repairs are even more difficult than those of arteries because the walls are far more friable and they clot more readily.

12

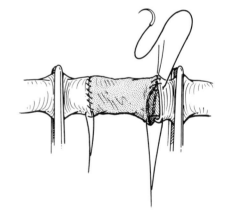

Vascular repairs may need to be protected with long fasciotomies (splitting the fascia under the skin), if there has been considerable delay in re-establishing arterial flow, so that the soft tissues can swell without impeding blood flow.

Nerves

Nerves should be debrided if they are obviously dead and badly torn, but no attempt should be made at initial debridement to carry out a repair. It is best merely to mark the ends of the cleaned nerve with a stainless steel clip or a small bit of metal suture, note their anatomic positions carefully and precisely in the record, and leave them for another time when a specialist in this area can achieve optimal operative reapproximation using an operating microscope under ideal conditions.

13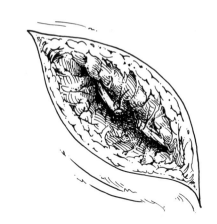

DRESSING THE TRAUMATIC WOUND: DELAYED PRIMARY CLOSURE

Experience on many battlefields has shown that the immediate or primary closure of contaminated traumatic wounds is a serious error and that infection is almost a certainty. Instead, the debrided wound should be dressed with an occlusive dressing and repaired by delayed primary closure under aseptic conditions four to five days after the injury.

Chapter 10 provides the details of delayed primary closure. The wound is first lined with a single layer of fine mesh gauze so that every area of tissue is covered. The entire cavity is then filled with fluffed-up gauze that, in turn, is covered with large absorbent pads. Next, the entire dressing is isolated from the environment with several occlusive layers of adhesive tape. *This dressing is not disturbed until the time of closure* unless there are signs of uncontrolled infection such as fever, an unusually foul odor, excessive pain, or a patient who is obviously not getting better. This occlusive dressing technique is described in detail in Chapter 18.

14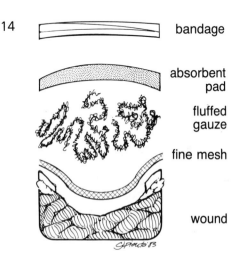

bandage

absorbent pad

fluffed gauze

fine mesh

wound

Delayed primary closure is performed in the operating room under sterile conditions, four to five days after the injury. If these amenities are not available, the nearest attainable approximation of these conditions should be used—namely, careful aseptic technique with mask and gloves and liberal use of local anesthesia. The closure should not be delayed much longer than the sixth day because that 48- to 72-hour interval appears to be a golden period when the best results can be obtained with the lowest incidence of infection. Contraindications to proceeding with the repair are an infected wound with inflammation or evidence of inadequate debridement with considerable remaining contamination. Such findings are rare in a well-debrided wound, and almost all traumatic wounds can be closed on the fourth or fifth day after injury.

The closure consists in excising just enough granulation tissue and a slim edge of skin to permit mobilization and gentle approximation of skin and soft tisues by a minimum number of gently tied 2-0 or 3-0 Prolene sutures.

15a

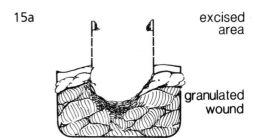

excised area

granulated wound

No drains are used. If the amount of remaining skin is not adequate, a thin split-thickness graft may be required to complete the coverage. A dry, small, sterile dressing will usually suffice after delayed primary closure. Infections are rare; if redness or purulence develops, removal of only one or two of the stitches usually suffices. Sutures after primary closure should usually be left in place for about two weeks to ensure complete healing.

15b

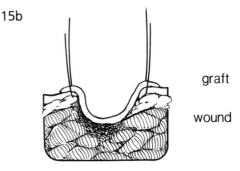

graft

wound

10 · *Principles of Wound Closure*

WALTER J. PORIES, M.D.

Wounds treated gently and closed precisely heal well with minimal scarring. A hairline scar documents the operator's skill; the public is not wrong to judge a surgeon's competence by the scars he or she leaves behind.

In contrast, rough treatment of wounds, with crushing of tissues, failure to achieve hemostasis, incomplete cleansing, and tightly drawn, strangulating sutures will lead to infection, breakdown, and unsightly, painful scars. The wound shown here will not heal well.

1

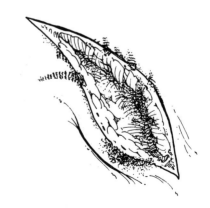

We discussed the importance of making incisions and carrying out excisions in the direction of the wrinkle lines in Chapter 4; the point deserves re-emphasis. Incisions parallel to wrinkle lines heal well, with minimal, almost invisible scars; incisions or wounds that cross these lines close with thick, broad, and unsightly scars.

For optimal healing, the wound should have fresh edges and be clean. Surgical incisions and simple lacerations can usually be closed directly, but many traumatic wounds require debridement (discussed in Chapter 9). In most old wounds excision of a *thin* margin of scar and granulations is indicated to afford mobility and to provide fresh healing surfaces.

2

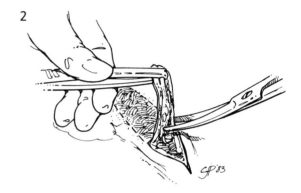

Prior to closure, all loose fat, clot, and other detritus should be picked up from the wound surfaces with a dry sponge.

3

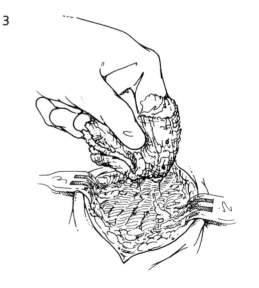

Copious irrigation with saline solution enhances wound cleanliness. The addition of 0.5 gm of kanamycin to 500 ml of the irrigating solution is a useful adjunct if contamination has been heavy.

4

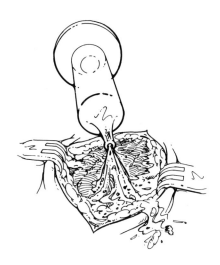

The well-prepared wound is red, clean, odorless, and remarkably pain free. Fresh, cleanly incised wounds heal best, but even badly contaminated wounds can heal nicely with minimal scarring if these basic principles are followed.

PRIMARY, SECONDARY, AND DELAYED CLOSURE

Wounds can be closed by primary intention, secondary intention, or delayed closure. Tissues that are clean and free of infection can be approximated by *primary closure*—that is, immediate repair with suture, to heal by primary intention. If the closure is well done, optimal healing and minimal scarring will follow.

5

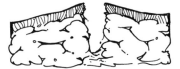

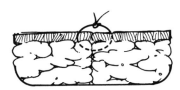

Wounds allowed to granulate through contamination, neglect, or other causes are said to undergo healing by *secondary intention*. The safety of this approach to infected wounds has been proven for centuries; its disadvantage is the long time required for healing and the heavy and often painful scarring that results. In addition, the wound never develops a good cover; the thick scar is only surfaced usually with a single layer of epithelium, which lacks the anchoring rete pegs, and it is thus easily wiped raw with even the slightest abrasion. In addition, the heavy scars may produce contractures and secondary deformities. Accordingly, wounds closed by secondary intention often require re-excision and even grafting to produce sound cosmetic and functional results.

6

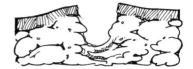

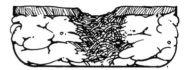

Delayed primary closure offers the advantages of secondary closure without its disadvantages. The method has been learned painfully during this century's wars and has saved innumerable lives over the last few decades. It is one of the great surgical advances. After the wound has been thoroughly cleansed and debrided (see Chapter 9), line it with a single layer of fine-mesh gauze and fill it with a bulky absorbent dressing, which is, in turn, isolated from the surrounding environment by several occlusive layers of adhesive tape. Do not disturb the wound for four to five days.

7

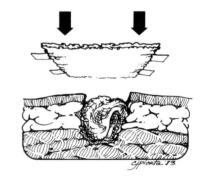

At the end of that period, uncover it under aseptic conditions. The wound can almost always be closed at that time with interrupted sutures of nylon or polypropylene. The scars produced by delayed primary closure are often as fine as those produced by immediate repair.

8

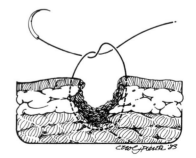

SUTURE TECHNIQUE

The principles of good suture technique include the anatomic layer-by-layer restoration of the injured tissues by a minimum number of approximating, but not strangling, sutures and the avoidance of dead space (empty pockets within the wound where the layers remain separated because of tension or lack of tissue); such dead space is soon filled with serum and liquefied fat, a ready target for infection.

Therefore, close wounds in layers: mucosa to mucosa, muscle to muscle, and skin to skin. We prefer to use absorbable suture materials such as 3-0 or 4-0 Vicryl or Dexon for the repair of mucosa and muscle and nonabsorbable suture such as nylon or polypropylene for critical fascial layers and skin. Muscle should be sutured in a single layer (as shown) only if the muscle is thin. If the muscle is thick, the sutures should be confined to the investing fascial layers because muscle, by itself, does not hold sutures and will merely necrose.

9

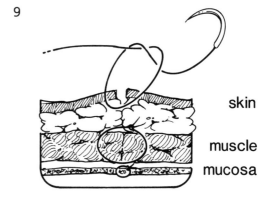

skin

muscle

mucosa

Sutures should be tied just tightly enough to bring the tissues into apposition. If tied too tightly, sutures will strangulate and cut through the tissues. Controlled approximation can be done most easily by tying a granny instead of a square knot (because this type of knot allows for controlled slippage), cinching it to just the right degree of tension, and then locking it in place with a squaring half-hitch. If a stitch is tied too tightly, cut it out and do it again instead of leaving it in place; otherwise, it will produce, at the least, excessive pain or, at worst, gangrene and infection.

Each suture is a foreign body and can therefore serve as a nidus for infection. Accordingly, use the least number of sutures possible, and trim all knots to short ends.

PROPERTIES OF VARIOUS SUTURE MATERIALS

Sutures vary greatly in their tissue reactivity and in their enhancement of infection. Monofilament sutures are much less likely to offer crevices for bacteria than braided sutures. Sutures made from organic materials such as catgut, silk, and cotton support bacterial growth and lead to infection much more readily than synthetic (nonorganic) sutures made of polyglycolic acid, nylon, polypropylene, and wire. Absorbable sutures produce more tissue reaction and inflammation than the nonabsorbable variety.

Sutures also vary in strength. Monofilament, nonabsorbable synthetic materials are the strongest; absorbable natural materials are the weakest. Strength varies with caliber; sutures are available in a broad variety of sizes from the massive #5 to the barely visible 12-0 filaments. For office surgery, the 3-0, 4-0, and 5-0 sizes meet most needs.

SELECTED SKIN CLOSURES

The *interrupted suture* remains the gold standard for wound closure because optimal healing will follow with minimal scarring if the sutures are precisely placed at a uniform level and tied gently. For the best cosmetic result in such areas as the face, the 5-0 Prolene sutures should be 1 mm apart and 1 mm from either edge; in other, less noticeable areas, interrupted sutures are usually placed 0.5 to 1 cm apart.

10

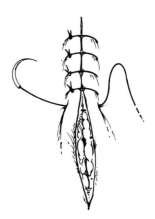

The *mattress suture* is useful if the skin is loose, as in clearly aged patients, and where precise coaptation of rather deep and irregular cuts is required. It is important that the stitches near the edge grasp less than 1 mm of tissue to avoid overlap.

11

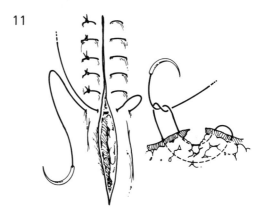

The *continuous running suture,* or baseball stitch, is a useful closure that can be created rapidly, producing excellent results if it is not pulled up tightly. It is particularly good for areas where the skin is thick, such as the back and thighs, and for emergency situations where numerous closures have to be made rapidly.

12

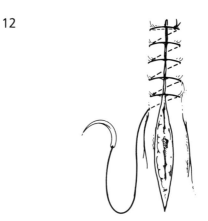

The *continuous mattress suture* has the combined advantages of the precision of the mattress suture and the speed of the continuous running stitch. Again, there is a danger of pulling the suture too tightly; this error must be carefully avoided.

13

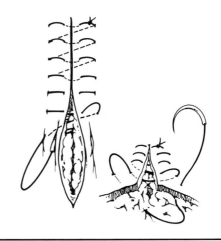

The *buried subcuticular suture* is a demanding stitch that is difficult to do well and requires some practice. A broiler chicken from the local supermarket offers excellent tissue for practice and can be eaten after the exercise! The stitch has two major advantages: it does not leave any railroad tracks, producing a fine and almost invisible hairline scar, and the sutures need not be removed later, a great advantage with children and with transient or anxious patients.

Begin the suture with a buried stitch in the far end of the wound. Bring the needle out exactly at the corner of the wound, and slide it lengthwise just below the surface of the skin at the junction between the dermis and epidermis (1 mm or less) in a series of stitches that always cross directly opposite each other across the wound.

16

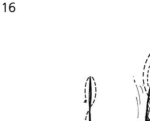
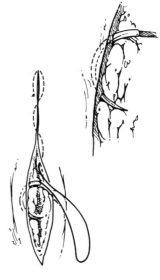

14

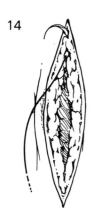

17

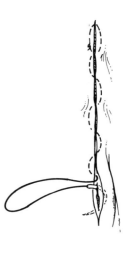

15

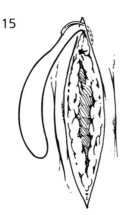

End the stitch by bringing it out at right angles to the wound, or anchor it by bringing it to the surface of the skin in line with the incision, and tie a small slipknot. Paint the wound with one or two layers of tincture of benzoin; when this adhesive material is dry, cover the wound with a Steri-strip while maintaining tension on the suture. Cut the suture flush with the bandage.

18

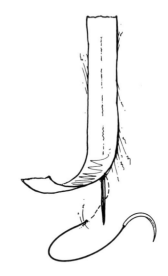

The *corner stitch* is useful for the repair of jagged lacerations and T-shaped incisions or injuries and can be used for the approximation of one or two corners. The suture is designed to avoid ischemic necrosis of corners, which commonly occurs in such injuries when repair with interrupted sutures cuts off the blood supply. The corner stitch is not difficult to learn and is extremely useful.

19

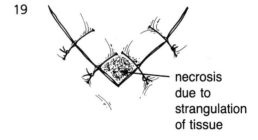

necrosis due to strangulation of tissue

The stitch begins on the side of the incision away from the corner, continues subcutaneously under the corner, entering and exiting at the same level, and reappears near its origin. It is tied just tightly enough to guide the corner into place.

20

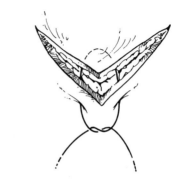

Similarly, T-shaped lacerations can be approxi-   21
mated in this fashion.

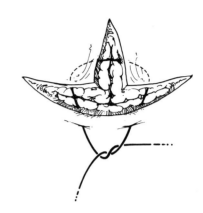

The *disposable skin stapler* is an efficient tool   22
for use when a large number of sutures are
needed to repair either long or multiple lacerations. The tissues are gently approximated with
fine-toothed forceps; one click of the stapler
then places the stitch. Skin stapling produces
excellent cosmetic results, and the staples are
easily removed with a specially designed device
that comes with the instrument. The only disadvantage is the expense of the stapler, but if
more than 20 sutures are required, it pays for
itself in time and effort.

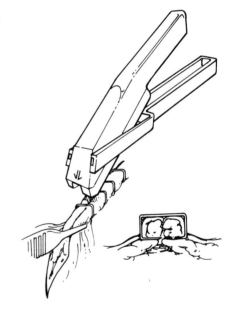

Microporous adhesive strips (Steri-strips, Ethi-strips) also offer an excellent means of approximation of small or superficial lacerations. The edges of the wound are painted with tincture of benzoin and allowed to dry. The edges are then gently pushed together with the fingers of one hand so that the other hand can apply the series of strips. The cosmetic results are excellent; the technique is particularly useful in small children and anxious adults.

23

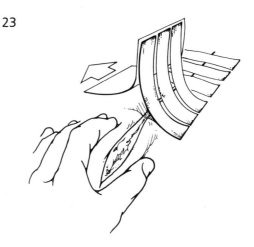

All these closures need only be covered with a light, dry dressing for a day or two unless longer coverage is wanted for cosmetic reasons. All patients must be instructed in the symptoms and signs of infection—namely, fever, pain, swelling, redness, and malaise—and should be told to report immediately to the physician if a complication is suspected. Usually only reassurance is required, but occasionally even the most minimal injuries or excisions can be followed by erysipelas, staphylococcal infection, and even gas gangrene or tetanus. A high degree of suspicion is an essential component of office surgery.

SUTURE REMOVAL

There are no firm rules about suture removal because there are variations in the rate of healing. In elderly, ill, diabetic, immunosuppressed patients and in those with cancer, for example, healing is slower than in the normal population. Even so, there are useful guidelines. In general, it is better to remove sutures earlier than later because of their tendency to leave railroad tracks, the small transverse scars that run the length of the wound and are often more unsightly than the main scar. The average time for suture removal depends on the vascularity of the tissues. Sutures can usually be removed according to the following schedule:

- Face, head, and neck: 3 days;

- Trunk: 7 days;

- Proximal extremities: 14 days;

- Distal extremities: 21 days.

These are obviously only guidelines; allowances have to be made for the needs of individual patients. If there is a question, leave the sutures in a few extra days or support the wound with Steri-strips after the sutures have been removed.

II · *Surgical Emergencies in Office Practice*

11 · *Emergency Procedures to Open the Airway*

WALTER J. PORIES, M.D. *and*
PAUL S. CAMNITZ, M.D.

The ABC rule for resuscitation reminds us that achieving an open airway is the first and most important step. A blocked pharynx and trachea can be opened by any of several techniques including manual clearing of the oral cavity and pharynx, placement of a plastic airway, insertion of endotracheal tubes, cricothyroidotomy, and tracheostomy, none of which is considered an office procedure. We describe these methods here, however, because they may be required in emergency or remote situations. Respiratory arrest can be a complication of local anesthesia in office surgery; airway compromise may occur in epiglottitis, croup, foreign body aspiration, angioneurotic edema, drug reactions, acciden-

tal extubation, and trauma to the larynx or trachea. The physician may have only a few minutes to avert disaster.

INITIAL PROCEDURES

The airway can be blocked by vomitus, aspirated dentures, or other material in the mouth and pharynx; by the tongue; or by a foreign body, such as an aspirated piece of meat, in the hypopharynx or supraglottic larynx. The first measures are aimed at clearing the pharynx, larynx, and respiratory tree:

Turn the head to one side and sweep the inside of the mouth and throat free of all material.

1

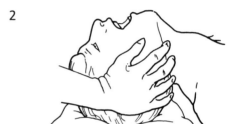

Return the chin to the midline, extend the neck, and lift the jaw upward, grasping it at the angle of the mandible. This action lifts the tongue from the posterior pharynx and opens the airway to the larynx.

2

Insert an airway by pressing the tongue caudad and upward with a tongue depressor or a finger and then sliding the airway in place. Do not twist or turn the airway, because such a maneuver can cause considerable mucosal damage; it is best to let the airway follow its natural curve. Usually it just drops into place almost by itself.

3

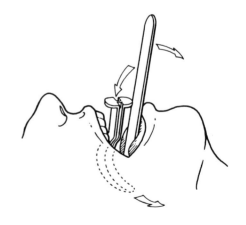

Begin ventilation with an Ambu bag or begin mouth-to-mouth respiration. Observe the thorax or, better, listen to both lungs to be certain that they are expanding.

4

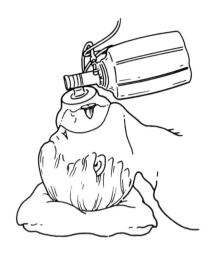

Unless the patient is expected to recover quickly, it is usually best to insert an endotracheal tube at this point for easier ventilation and cleansing of the respiratory tree.

If the lungs do not expand, there is probably an obstruction in either the larynx or the trachea. Such a foreign body can sometimes be removed by a finger hooking deep into the throat, by the Heimlich maneuver, or by a sharp slap on the patient's back. If these maneuvers are unsuccessful, proceed promptly with a cricothyroidotomy.

ENDOTRACHEAL INTUBATION USING THE LARYNGOSCOPE

Endotracheal intubation is not difficult if the head is positioned properly, the laryngoscope is well lighted and fitted with the appropriate blade, and the operator remains calm and takes time to obtain a clear view of the structures.

Laryngoscopy can be performed with either a straight or a curved blade. The straight blade is designed to extend beyond the epiglottis and lift it out of the way; the curved blade is placed anterior to the epiglottis and into the vallecula

The endotracheal tube should be as large as possible (a #8 is a good size for most adults) and equipped with a large low-pressure balloon. If there is time, check the balloon for leaks and test the suction before beginning intubation.

Extend the head so that the mouth, pharynx, and larynx are aligned along an axis.

5

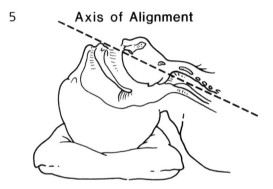

Axis of Alignment

Hold the laryngoscope in your left hand, insert the blade through the left side of the mouth, and aim toward the midline. If you are using the straight blade, lift up the epiglottis to expose the vocal cords and the trachea.

6

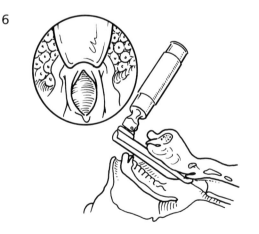

If you are using the curved blade, insert it through the left side, aim toward the midline, and lift up the base of the tongue just in front of the epiglottis to expose the larynx and trachea.

7

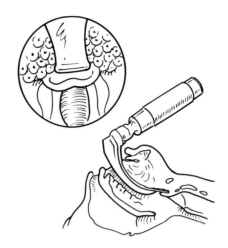

Insinuate the tube gently between the cords and inflate the balloon just enough to seal the trachea.

8

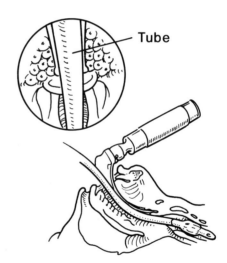

Tube

Connect the endotracheal tube to the Ambu bag, and liberally ventilate the patient. Attach the oxygen line to the base of the Ambu bag. As soon as the patient has been well ventilated, clean out the tracheobronchial tree with the suction catheter. Suctioning is dangerous because it can cause serious anoxia and arrhythmias; it should therefore be done in brief pulses well separated by intervals of vigorous ventilation. A good rule is to hold your own breath while you are suctioning the patient. When you are short of breath, the patient is seriously anoxic and needs to be ventilated promptly.

9

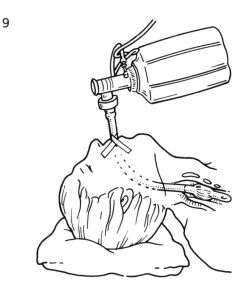

BLIND ENDOTRACHEAL INTUBATION

Dr. Jack Welch, professor and chairman of our department of anesthesia, developed and continues to employ a rapid method of laryngeal intubation that eliminates use of the laryngoscope and its many attendant problems. He opens the airway by precise positioning of the head and neck and then guides the endotracheal tube by feel into the trachea. He has performed more than 10,000 of these intubations without a significant complication, even in patients presenting difficult anatomic challenges. The technique is easily mastered, and he has had little difficulty teaching it to our medical students. Once you learn it, you'll use a laryngoscope only rarely.

The blind method seems to be associated with much less mucosal and dental damage than other methods and is particularly helpful in patients whose head cannot be extended. The method should be used with caution in patients with hoarseness, dysphonia, or tumors; in such patients it is safer to inspect the cords and the pathway of the tube before intubation.

Insert a metal stylet into the endotracheal tube to stiffen it; be sure that the stylet does not protrude beyond the tip. Test the balloon and lubricate the tube thoroughly.

10

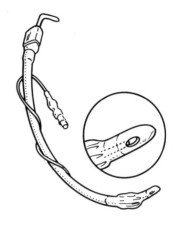

Lift the chin firmly by grasping the anterior mandible in the midline, using thumb and index finger.

11

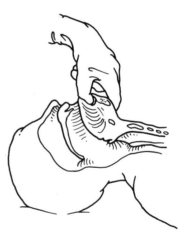

Insinuate the tube precisely in the midline with the delicacy of a safecracker, being guided by feel and the absence of resistance. If the tube meets an obstruction in the midline, it is probably the epiglottis; if the obstruction is to either side, it is probably the pyriform sinus.

12

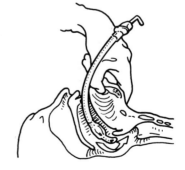

The thyroid cartilage is a critical landmark. It will deviate if the tube is misdirected but will remain in the midline as long as the intubation proceeds properly.

13

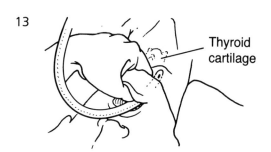

Thyroid cartilage

Similarly, a bulge on either side of the neck is an indication that the tip of the tube has been lodged in either pyriform sinus; it must be redirected into the midline.

In short, if you meet resistance you are probably impinging on the epiglottis or either pyriform sinus. Back up, be certain that you are in the midline, and advance again, working your way under the epiglottis.

14

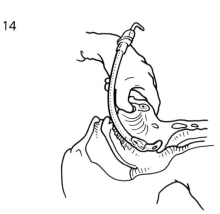

The tube can enter either the esophagus or the trachea but will almost always enter the trachea if the tip is pointed upward as it is advanced. The tactile sensations differ according to whether the tube is in the trachea or in the esophagus; in the esophagus the tube moves with a sticky sensation; in the trachea it gives and then drops in effortlessly with a loss of resistance.

Connect the tube to an Ambu bag, inflate the balloon, and listen to both lungs to be certain that the tube is correctly placed. Initiate active ventilation, and, when oxygenaton is adequate, cleanse the tube and the airway with endotracheal suction.

COMPLICATIONS OF ENDOTRACHEAL INTUBATION

Serious complications can occur with either method of intubation, including the following:

Gastric dilation is particularly common if several attempts have been required to place the tube. The dilated stomach can be perforated, can interfere with diaphragmatic excursion, and can produce long-term ileus, emesis, and aspiration. Insert a nasogastric tube at once if there is any suspicion that the stomach has been blown up with air.

If the endotracheal tube is inserted too deeply, it will block the left main-stem bronchus. Check the ventilation of both sides with a stethoscope and a chest roentgenogram immediately after intubation; if breath sounds are diminished on the left, pull back the tube until it is above the carina and breath sounds can be heard clearly.

Other complications include nasal necrosis, epistaxis, hoarseness from injury to the vocal cords, and obstruction of the tube by inspissated secretions.

CRICOTHYROIDOTOMY

Cricothyroidotomy is an elegantly simple and safe emergency procedure that is far safer than a tracheostomy in an emergency. It is not as good as peroral tracheal intubation, which can, of course, be done even more quickly and more safely, but in instances of pharyngeal or laryngeal obstruction, it is the procedure of choice. Cricothyroidotomy does not replace tracheostomy, a difficult procedure carried out for long-term endotracheal intubation.

The cricothyroid membrane is the site chosen because there are no important organs between the skin and the airway that can be damaged, there are no major vessels in this area, the airway is relatively close to the skin, the airway is protected only by a thin membrane anteriorly, and the airway is shielded posteriorly by the cricoid cartilage, a protection against inadvertent perforation through the airway into the esophagus.

15

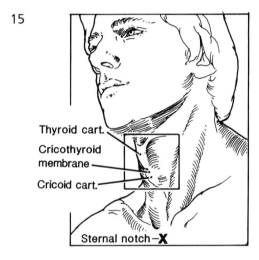

Thyroid cart.
Cricothyroid membrane
Cricoid cart.
Sternal notch—**X**

16

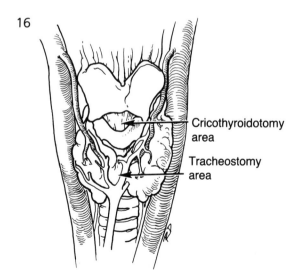

Cricothyroidotomy area

Tracheostomy area

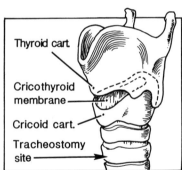

Thyroid cart.
Cricothyroid membrane
Cricoid cart.
Tracheostomy site

Place a roll under the shoulders and hyperextend the neck. If there is time, wash the neck with antiseptic solution. Identify the anatomic landmarks. Identify the cricothyroid membrane; it lies immediately under the skin between the thyroid and cricoid cartilages. Feel the high sharp bump made by the edge of the thyroid and cricoid cartilages, and follow it caudad; the first indentation is the right spot.

17

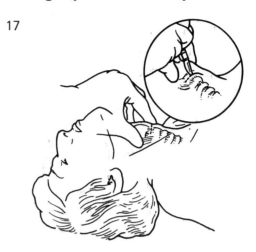

Steady the larynx (the thyroid cartilage) between the thumb and forefinger of the left hand and infiltrate the area (if the patient is still conscious) with 1% lidocaine and epinephrine. Puncture the skin and the cricothyroid membrane exactly in the midline, pointing the scalpel transversely. Extend the incision 1 cm toward each side.

Insert the Delaborde dilator and slide in the endotracheal tube just enough so that the balloon can no longer be seen. Inflate the balloon only to stop the air leak when the lungs are inflated. If a Delaborde dilator is not available (check a tracheostomy set; one is almost always there), a Kelly clamp will serve almost as well.

18

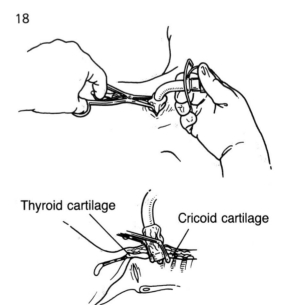

Thyroid cartilage

Cricoid cartilage

Bleeding is unusual with this procedure and is best avoided by staying strictly in the midline and not extending the incision too far to either side.

In some cases requiring cricothyroidotomy, the physician must use whatever tools are at hand. Some emergency rooms have cricothyroidotomy cannulas, which are useful, but they are not usually immediately at hand. Insertion of large-bore needles or intravenous catheters allows one to deliver either mouth-to-needle resuscitation or oxygen directly to the needle.

The procedure is still under evaluation. Although some have reported as many as 655 cricothyroidotomies with only 40 minor complications, others have had difficulties with later strictures and serious laryngeal pathology. There is little question, however, that cricothyroidotomy is the best emergency procedure for airway obstruction when endotracheal intubation cannot be done. At present, the long-term effects of cricothyroidotomy are unknown. The cricothyroidotomy should be withdrawn as soon as feasible and replaced with a peroral or transnasal endotracheal tube or an orthodox tracheostomy.

EMERGENCY TRACHEOSTOMY

Tracheostomy is not really an office procedure. It is much more difficult and far less safe than a cricothyroidotomy. Even so, we do include it on the grounds that this reference for office surgical procedures may be the only one available to a physician at a remote site. If at all possible, when doing a tracheostomy, make it an elective procedure. Tracheostomy is best performed with an endotracheal tube in place, al-lowing the operator to work in an unhurried and deliberate manner. Tracheostomies are technically very difficult, especially in children; in some series in children, mortality has been as high as 50% from catastrophic mishaps such as torn carotid arteries, severed tracheas, cut recurrent laryngeal nerves, and uncontrollable venous hemorrhage. Tracheostomies are also technically difficult in obese patients and patients with deformed or fixed cervical spines. In short, tracheostomies are not the simple, quick, emergency procedures they are purported to be, and they are best avoided if at all possible.

Before beginning a tracheostomy, read these directions with care and, in particular, be certain that all the required equipment is available and functioning. The tracheostomy tube and its balloon should be tested; if at all possible, a second one should be available, in case the first is dropped or does not work properly. A reliable way to check for leaks is to blow up the balloon and its connections under water; air bubbles indicate a leaky, defective tube.

Place a rolled towel under the patient's shoulders and extend his or her neck to pull the trachea out of the thorax as far as possible. This position is contraindicated, however, in patients with epiglottitis or croup, as laying them down may precipitate total laryngeal obstruction. If there is time, wash the area thoroughly with an antiseptic.

Next, palpate landmarks. Locate the sternal notch, the cricoid cartilage, and the inferior border of the thyroid cartilage. Occasionally one can feel the trachea and the thyroid gland.

If the patient is still conscious, infiltrate the area with 1% lidocaine with epinephrine as far down as the trachea.

Make a 2- to 3-in midline incision upward from the sternal notch. This will leave an unsightly scar, but it will also avoid time-consuming attention to laterally located vessels. In non-emergency tracheostomies we use transverse incisions because we then have time enough to handle the large veins often encountered in such an incision. Scars can always be revised later.

19   Midline incision
     —neck hyperextended

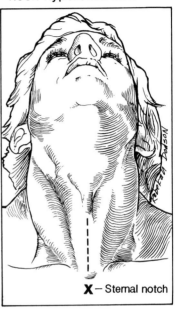

X – Sternal notch

20

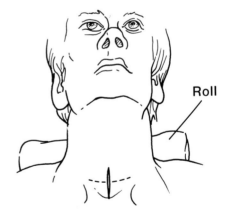

Roll

Extend the incision to the strap muscles, which always lie deeper than one expects. The strap muscles can be identified by their salmon-red color.

21

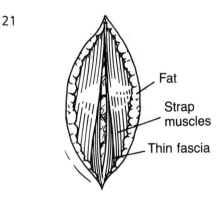

Fat

Strap muscles

Thin fascia

Spread the strap muscles in the midline with a large clamp. This step is often difficult. The strap muscles are often fused in the midline and are occasionally covered by a network of troublesome veins. Such veins can sometimes be separated in the midline but occasionally must be divided and ligated.

22

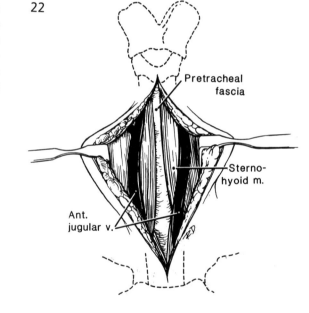

Pretracheal fascia

Sterno-hyoid m.

Ant. jugular v.

Guide each step by feeling often with the finger. We cannot emphasize too much how easy it is to get away from the midline, especially if an anxious assistant is retracting too enthusiastically. Always aim for the midline of the trachea.

If you are fortunate, the trachea will come into view directly under the strap muscles. It is more common, however, to encounter the thyroid gland and its generous blood supply. If this is the case, try to push the thyroid upward to expose the trachea and, if possible, extend the incision farther toward the sternal notch. If this does not provide the needed exposure, you may have to divide the thyroid gland with clamps and ligatures, a most difficult procedure.

23

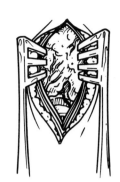

When the trachea is brought into view, aspiration of air with a small-bore needle will assure the surgeon that the trachea is indeed the structure identified. This is particularly important in children in whom the rings have not yet calcified. After the trachea is exposed, it is helpful to apply traction and elevate it into view. Constant control is needed as well, in case immediate access is necessary. The surgeon can accomplish both of these goals in two ways. One way is to place two heavy stitches through the second or third tracheal ring on either side of the midline; these sutures can be left in place after the tube is secured to provide easy access in the event of dislodgement.

24

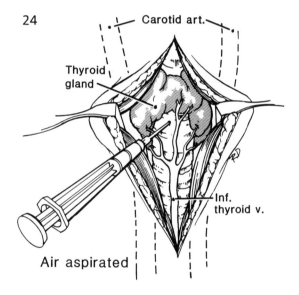

Carotid art.

Thyroid gland

Inf. thyroid v.

Air aspirated

25

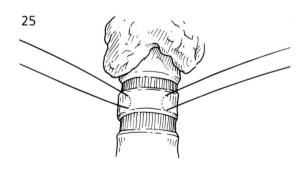

A second method of securing the trachea is by use of a cricoid hook, a standard instrument on tracheostomy trays; this hook is placed just below the cricoid cartilage and pulled cephalad.

26

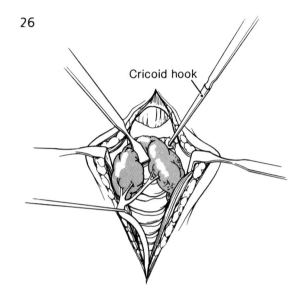

Cricoid hook

Various incisions can be employed to enter the trachea. One can cut a window into the second tracheal ring approximately 5 to 8 mm in the horizontal plane and one ring long in the vertical plane. This method has several advantages: it establishes an airway before the tube is in, reduces the incidence of fragmented cartilage, and allows easy re-establishment of the airway in case of accidental dislodgement. The disadvantage is that occasionally granulation tissue will grow to the window after decannulation, causing subglottic stenosis.

27

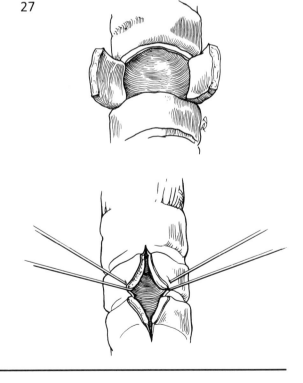

A better choice is an incision approximately 3/4 in long in the midline opening the second and third tracheal rings.

28

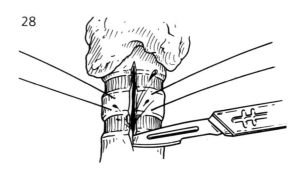

Be prepared for a messy spurt of air, sputum, and blood; have the suction catheter ready. This incision is particularly good for children since it avoids injury to the recurrent laryngeal nerves. In adults, these paired nerves run posteriorly in the tracheoesophageal groove; in children, however, they are more anterior, along the tracheal wall. A midline vertical incision will avoid injury to them. For added safety, the edges of the tracheal incision may be sutured to the skin. A third type of incision, the one most frequently used in adults, creates two laterally based flaps. Two incisions approximately 1 cm long are made, one below, the second above the second tracheal ring. These two incisions are connected in the midline, and the flaps are retracted outward so that the tracheostomy tube can be placed between them. A dilator is usually not necessary.

29

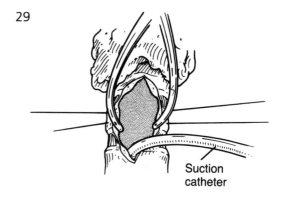

Suction catheter

Insert the endotracheal tube far enough to conceal the top of the balloon.

30

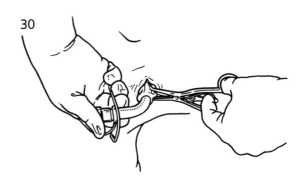

Inflate the balloon just sufficiently to stop the leakage of air from the trachea. Make sure, when placing a tracheostomy tube, that it is in the trachea and not alongside it in the mediastinum. After the tracheostomy is done, the surgeon must make sure the tip of the tube is not resting on the carina or in a main-stem bronchus.

31

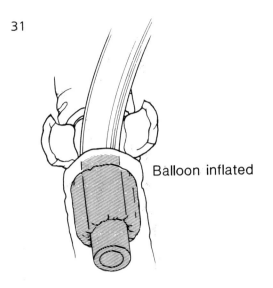

Balloon inflated

32

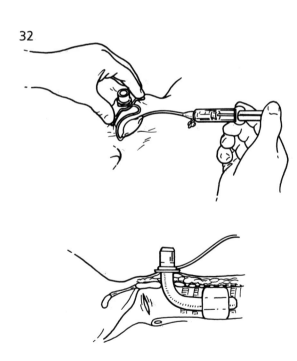

Do not close the incision with sutures. Leave it open to drain so that any bleeding can be detected quickly and stopped. If the wound were to be tightly closed, frequently subcutaneous air would spread throughout the neck. The tube should be secured with tracheostomy tapes around the neck.

33

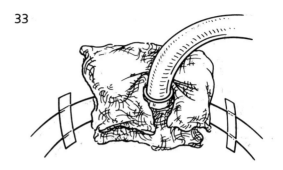

Finally, send the patient to a hospital as quickly as possible.

Additional mention should be made about the changing of tracheostomy tubes. Usually after five days there is an excellent tract from the skin to the trachea, allowing easy access, in which case there is little problem regarding tube changes. Should the patient have an early failure of the balloon system, however, immediate replacement of the tube will be necessary for adequate ventilation. When the tube is thus removed early, the swollen and inflamed tissues of the neck may cover the opening into the trachea, particularly when the thyroid isthmus has not been divided. To diminish the potential for disaster, the surgeon should insert a suction catheter through the tracheostomy tube into the trachea. The tracheostomy tube can then be removed over the catheter, which serves as a guide for the new tracheostomy tube. This precaution both permits sure access to the trachea and, if necessary, can accommodate emergency short-term ventilation.

34

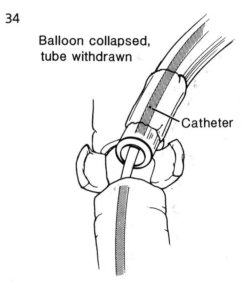

Balloon collapsed, tube withdrawn

Catheter

12 · *Venous and Arterial Access*

WALTER J. PORIES, M.D.

The family physician should have a number of approaches available for rapid access to veins and arteries, especially if office surgery and the care of emergencies are a part of the practice. Therefore, for reference, this chapter includes some procedures that are not appropriate for most office practices but that may prove useful in remote or emergency situations.

It is important that the stage be set fully before a vascular access procedure is begun. One feels terribly helpless, after the artery or vein has been entered flawlessly, to find that the IV bottles have not been connected to the IV sets and

frustrated when an infective phlebitis develops the next day because of inadequate asepsis. It is good practice, therefore, to preview the procedure to be certain that all required materials are available and ready to function.

INSERTION OF AN INTRAVENOUS LINE

Insertion of an IV line is, admittedly, a procedure familiar to physicians. We include it in this chapter as the most common route of vascular access, with instructions that may be useful to paramedical personnel.

The first step in any vascular access procedure is preparation of the fluid and the tubing to be connected to the needle of the cannula. Check the bottle to *be certain that the solution is the correct one and that it contains no sediment.*

1

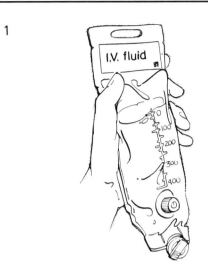

Break the seal and connect the set without contaminating either the stylet or the diaphragm at the mouth of the bottle. If either of these is touched, it must be thoroughly cleansed with an antiseptic before being used.

2a

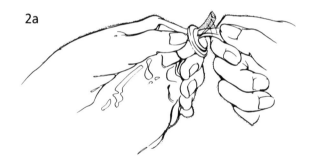

2b

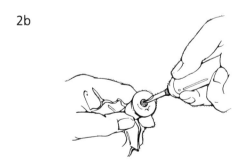

Hang the bottle and allow the system to fill by gravity. Squeeze the drip chamber enough to fill it about halfway and let the fluid run freely through the tubing until all air has cleared the system.

3a

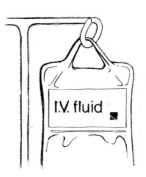

3b

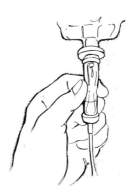

3c

The purpose of the IV line dictates its characteristics. If the intent is to provide a line for the treatment of shock, a large-bore cannula, at least a #18, should be placed; if the purpose is merely short-term restoration of lost fluids or administration of a medication, a short #22 needle will suffice; if the patient is a tiny infant, a #24 butterfly placed in a scalp vein may be adequate.

In adults, a #18 plastic cannula will serve for most situations. The bore, while large enough to permit administration of blood, is small enough for insertion into most peripheral veins without significant discomfort and without occluding the lumina, which would produce thrombosis. We prefer to use the plastic cannula rather than the bare needle because the sharp tip of the needle is often painful and can perforate the vein, causing infiltration. In contrast, insertion of plastic cannulas is usually painless, and perforation is rare.

After the tourniquet has been applied, the veins can be filled by having the patient flex his or her fist. The most peripheral veins should be used initially to save the more proximal veins for later. If the vessels are difficult to find or if they are in spasm, they will usually distend with time, with gentle digital tapping, or by application of heat or an irritant such as alcohol.

4

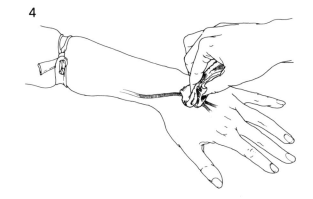

The site is thoroughly cleansed with an alcohol or Betadine swab. This should not be merely a perfunctory act; the skin should be scrubbed fairly vigorously and then not contaminated again during the procedure. Contaminated peripheral IVs produce dangerous bacteremias that can infect prostheses, cause subacute bacterial endocarditis, and induce purulent phlebitis.

Local anesthesia is not normally needed for #18 or smaller needles. For larger needles, however, and for anxious patients, the considerate physician will infiltrate the site first with 1 to 2 ml of 1% lidocaine.

The vein is stabilized by traction with one hand, while the other hand pushes the needle with its cannula into the vessel.

5

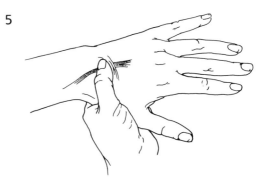

The cannulation is most likely to be successful if the needle is new, if the bevel faces upward, and if it enters the skin at 45 degrees and spears the vein at an angle of about 15 degrees.

6

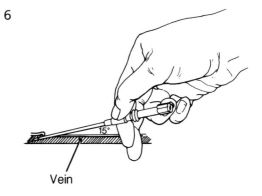

Vein

Blood should appear in the plastic cap of the
needle, or "flashback" should occur when the
stylet is pulled back if the vein has been entered.
The needle is then gently advanced within the
lumen for another 3 to 5 mm to be certain that
it is inside the vessel. Many practitioners prefer
to maintain suction with a small syringe during
the insertion, but we believe that this makes
manipulation of the needle difficult and wastes
a syringe as well.

7

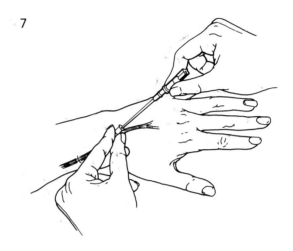

8

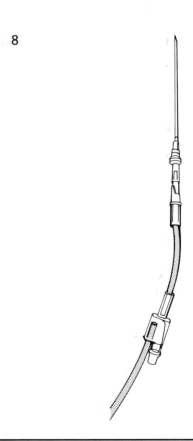

The plastic cannula is then advanced until its hub is flush with the skin, and the tourniquet is released. The needle is removed and the plastic cannula is connected to the IV connecting set routinely, to permit addition of medications or flushing of the apparatus without disturbing the IV dressing. The tourniquet is removed, and flow is begun by opening the IV control valve.

A small mound of antibiotic ointment is placed on the cannula where it enters the skin. The hub is then taped firmly in place, and the area is covered with an occlusive dressing. Arm boards are usually not needed for cooperative adults if cannulas are used instead of needles.

9

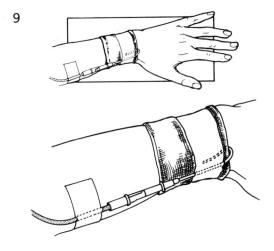

In newborn infants and small children, veins are more difficult to find but can usually be located on the back of the hand, the dorsum of the foot, and the scalp. Veins of the scalp are particularly useful in small infants; they can usually be distended by shaving a small area of overlying skin. Small butterfly needles, #21 and #23, serve well; the plastic wings aid greatly in the manipulation of the needle and offer a good surface for anchoring strips of tape. In small children, IV lines must be well anchored; arm boards or other restraints will usually be needed to protect the system.

10

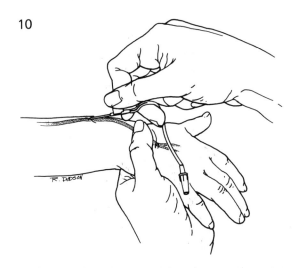

IV lines should be removed or relocated if there is evidence of local or unexplained systemic infection, thrombosis, or infiltration. If infection is the reason for the removal, the tip of the cannula should be sent for culture.

The IV is removed by gently releasing all of the tape from the skin and then withdrawing the cannula from the vein and skin. A Band-Aid usually suffices for a dressing. A brief period of pressure may be required to control bleeding if the IV has been in place for only a short period.

PERCUTANEOUS INSERTION OF A LONG CANNULA

Long, large-bore cannulas (#16 or larger) placed so that they empty into the atrium are useful for administration of large volumes of blood, measurement of central venous pressures, and infusion of materials such as nutrients or chemotherapeutic agents, which require rapid venous mixing and high flow if thrombosis is to be avoided.

A large vein is selected with the help of a tourniquet, and the overlying skin is infiltrated gently with several milliliters of 1% lidocaine through a #25 needle. The area is massaged to diffuse the anesthetic agent, allowing time for it to become effective.

The vein is stabilized by applying traction on the skin. The vessel is then punctured with the needle's bevel facing upward and entering the vein at an angle of about 15 degrees. Blood will appear in the cannula if the vein has been cannulated properly. The tourniquet is then released.

11

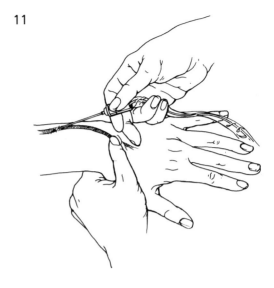

The cannula is advanced into the vein by pushing the catheter within its plastic sheath while stabilizing the hub of the needle. When the cannula is in, the needle is fully withdrawn from the skin and the hub of the cannula is fastened to the hub of the needle. The plastic sheath is then removed.

12

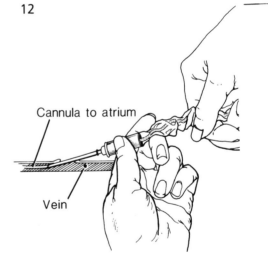

Cannula to atrium

Vein

The needle tip protector is applied to prevent damage to the plastic cannula by the sharp tip of the needle, a small dollop of Betadine ointment is applied, the apparatus is taped securely in place, and the infusion is begun.

13

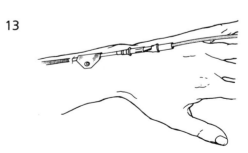

VENOUS CUTDOWN

There is often too great a reluctance to use venous cutdowns. If done properly, they provide rapid venous access with minimal discomfort and scar.

The site is selected by filling the veins using a tourniquet. If a vein is wider than 3 mm and is not thrombosed, it can usually be cannulated. If no suitable veins can be found in the upper extremity or if the need for access is urgent, the saphenous vein should be used at the ankle because it can be located easily in the groove just in front of the medial malleolus.

In adults, we prefer cannulas in the range of #18 to #12 but usually settle for a #18 to minimize the chances for thrombosis. In infants we most commonly use a #22, and in most children we use a #18 or #20.

The proposed incision, which needs to be only slightly longer than the width of the vein, is precisely outlined using a thin permanent-ink marker, and the outline is allowed to dry.

14

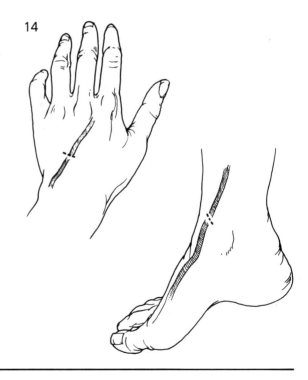

15

The area is cleansed thoroughly with an antiseptic agent and infiltrated with 5 ml of 1% lidocaine with epinephrine through a #25 needle. The skin is then gently massaged until the anesthetic agent has been absorbed and the normal contour of the tissues restored.

An incision of 0.5 to 1 cm (no longer) is made directly over the vein into the fat.

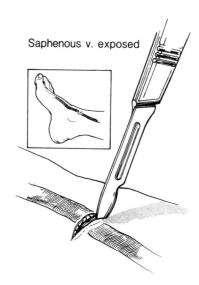

Saphenous v. exposed

16

Small mosquito forceps are used to spread the tissues in the direction of the vein until the vein is well exposed.

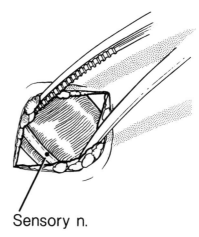

Sensory n.

The forceps are then turned to lift the vein into the wound. Occasionally, and especially in the saphenous area, a small sensory nerve is attached to the vein. This small fiber should be gently separated from the vein by another forceps and allowed to drop back into the wound. This is an important step because a ligated nerve can cause considerable discomfort.

A tie of 4-0 silk or one of the absorbable synthetic sutures is passed under the vein by grasping the vein or the tie in the middle and cutting the loop after it has been passed. This technique eliminates passing two ties separately.

17

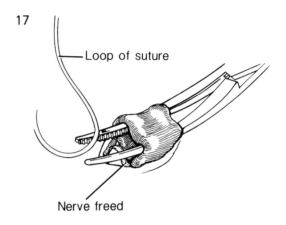

Loop of suture

Nerve freed

The distal tie is tied. The ends of the tie are left long and grasped with a clamp to help provide traction. The proximal tie is lifted gently to bring the vein into the wound, and a small cut is made with the tips of the iris scissors or similar small, sharp scissors.

18a

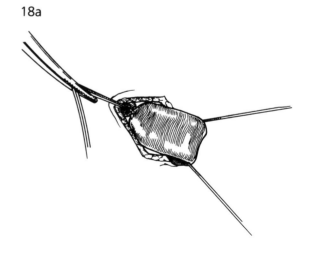

18b

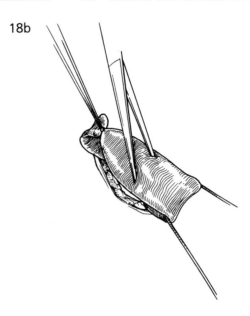

The cannula can usually be inserted easily, but if there is difficulty, the tip of the catheter can be beveled for easier introduction. A plastic cannula inserter, which looks like a tiny grooved director, can be useful, especially for small children. Cannula inserters are inexpensive and worth having available; with difficult vessels they can make the impossible task easy.

19

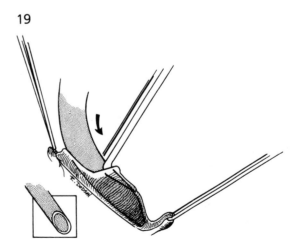

Healing will be best and the chances for infection will be minimized if the cannula is brought in through a separate puncture near the wound, but this is not essential.

20

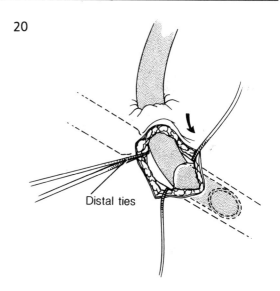

Distal ties

When the cannula has been advanced fully, the proximal tie is fastened snugly around the vein and its contained plastic tubing. The cannula is then connected to an IV connecting set, which, in turn, is attached to the IV tubing and a container of the appropriate solution.

21

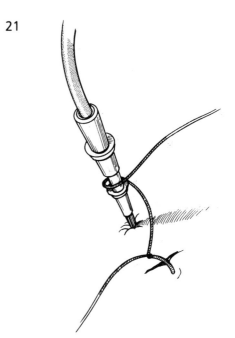

The wound usually can be approximated with one suture; if it takes more than two, the incision is probably too long. The end of that suture can be used to hold the cannula in place by tying it about the needle at the hub. The lines are taped securely.

The wound is dressed with a dollop of antibiotic ointment and covered with an occlusive dressing. The dressing is changed under sterile conditions every 48 hr or more frequently if it becomes soiled or shows signs of infection.

PERCUTANEOUS CANNULATION OF THE SUBCLAVIAN VEIN

Percutaneous cannulation of the subclavian vein (insertion of a subclavian line) is a difficult technique and should be practiced initially in the presence of an experienced observer. Once learned, however, it is a most useful method for gaining rapid and safe access to a large vein, especially in a critically ill patient.

Even in the best of hands, however, serious complications can occur because the needles used for subclavian punctures are large and sharp and can cause considerable damage. A lateral pass can make a large tear in either the subclavian vein or artery, producing massive hemorrhage into the tissues or the pleural space. Such bleeding is doubly dangerous because it may be difficult to recognize in a patient already in distress. Similarly, the apex of the lung can be torn, producing a pneumothorax or, worse, a tension pneumothorax. Another complication is the consequence of the cannula's perforating the wall of the distal vein: the infusions fail to enter the circulation and, instead, pour into the pleural space; thus, the patient's fluid volume is not expanded, and the patient is further compromised by the development of a restricting hydrothorax or hemothorax.

Other less common complications include air embolism (caused by suction of air into the venous system when the system has been left open to the atmosphere), subclavian vein thrombosis, infection, misdirection of the catheter into the jugular vein, embolism of pieces of the catheter (caused by damage to the catheter by the needle edge), and myocardiac puncture, with or without hemopericardium and cardiac tamponade.

In spite of this frightening list, subclavian lines are used widely with few complications and with great benefit to patients. Experience has shown that the following guidelines can sharply reduce the incidence of mishaps:

- Complications lessen with experience. The first 10 to 15 insertions of subclavian cannulas should be supervised by someone with considerable experience.

- Abandon the procedure after two unsuccessful attempts.

- Whether the procedure is successful or not, it should be followed immediately by a roentgenogram of the chest to rule out complications and to check the position of the catheter.

- Positive pressure ventilation increases the chance for laceration of the lung. During insertion of a subclavian cannula, the patient should be taken off the ventilator and supported by manual methods, which are stopped during the actual puncture.

- Arteries pulsate. Withdraw the needle if pulsations are felt.

- Advance the cannula gently; if it doesn't move easily, it is either wrongly directed or is about to perforate the wall of the vein.

- The system must remain closed to the atmosphere because the negative pressure in the great veins (-5 cm) can suck in air and cause air embolism, filling the heart with foam. Disconnections and connections should be planned and performed quickly and should not take more than a fraction of a second. (Air embolism can be diagnosed by "squishy" heart sounds and a sharp fall in pressure; treatment should be the immediate placement of the patient in a steep head-down position with the right side elevated to force the foam out of the ventricles.)

- Be careful of the edge of the needle; it can damage the catheter and cause it to fragment and embolize.

- Observe sterile technique and guard the system carefully against infection. With good care, subclavian lines have been kept functioning for months without difficulty; with neglect, serious infections can follow within a day or two.

- Suspicion pays off. Never trust Mother Nature.

The patient ideally is supine for percutaneous cannulation of the subclavian vein, in a 10-20 Trendelenburg position, with the head turned to the opposite side and the arm close to the body. Some sources also recommend that a roll be placed under the shoulders to extend the neck. With experience, however, these requirements become less obligatory, and most of the central lines placed in our institution are inserted with the patient in the position required for that patient's care; if both arms are spread out and if the patient is flat on a backboard, even with the head somewhat elevated, members of the house staff still usually slide the lines

22

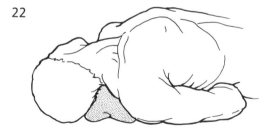

in easily. The main clues seem to be experience and careful attention to the anatomic relationships about the clavicle and the first rib (shown in the figure).

23

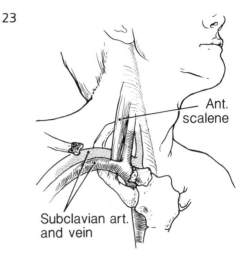

The skin is infiltrated with about 5 ml of 1% lidocaine and epinephrine in an area 2 to 3 cm below and just beyond the midpoint of the clavicle.

24

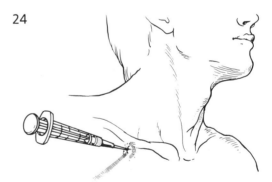

Insert the cannulation needle, sealed with a non-Luer-lock syringe, into the center of the anesthetized area, and direct it toward the suprasternal notch.

25

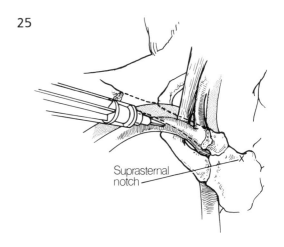

Suprasternal notch

Aimed properly, the needle will enter the subclavian vein in the angle formed between the upper surface of the first rib and the clavicle. If pulsations are felt, the needle is near the artery and should be withdrawn.

26

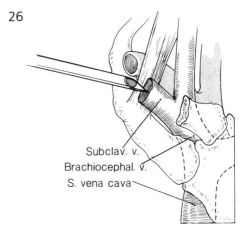

Subclav. v.
Brachiocephal. v.
S. vena cava

If the vein has been entered properly, blood should return easily upon gentle aspiration with the syringe. The bevel is then turned anteriorly and caudally, and the aspiration is repeated. If good flow continues, the syringe is removed and the hub of the needle is covered with a finger to prevent bleeding or the aspiration of air. The cannula is then introduced through the needle into the vena cava (a distance of about 13 to 15 cm in the adult). The advancement may be facilitated by turning the head back toward the midline or to the side of the punc-

27

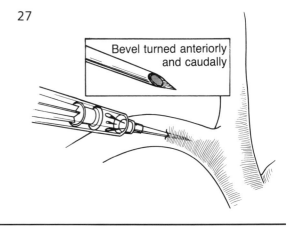

Bevel turned anteriorly and caudally

ture; if resistance is met, the catheter should not be advanced but should be pulled back 5 to 6 cm before another try is made.

28

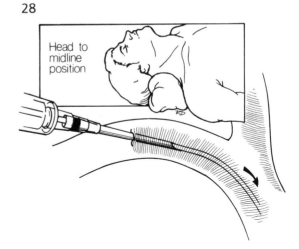

The needle is withdrawn and the needle and the cannula hubs are locked together. The aspiration is repeated to ensure that the system is functioning.

29

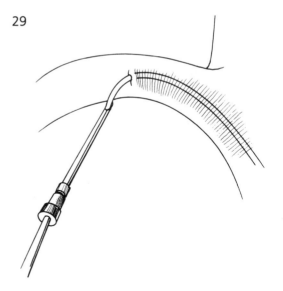

The cannula is attached to the IV and flushed with saline to prevent clotting. The cannula and its hub are fastened to the skin with a nonabsorbable suture such as silk or nylon. The entry site is protected with an antibiotic ointment and a carefully applied sterile occlusive dressing. A roentgenogram of the chest is made to assess the placement of the catheter and to rule out the presence of complications.

The external jugular and internal jugular veins can be cannulated by a similar procedure. These vessels are often easier to enter than the subclavian vein but are harder to anchor and keep in place because of the movements of the head.

INSERTION OF A SWAN-GANZ CATHETER

The insertion of a Swan-Ganz catheter is clearly not a procedure designed for the family physician's office, and its description is included in this chapter with considerable hesitation. The technique is virtually the same, however, as the one just described for the insertion of central venous lines. In addition, catheters of the Swan-Ganz type are being used so commonly in emergency rooms and critical care units that the family physician should be familiar with the technique of insertion, interpretation of results, and complications that might be encountered.

30

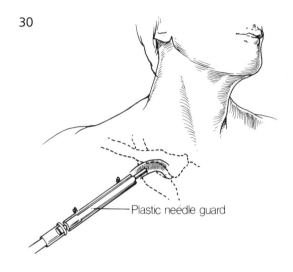
Plastic needle guard

The most commonly used variation of the Swan-Ganz catheter is the thermodilution type with a distal port (a) for measuring pulmonary artery and wedge pressures. The balloon holds 1 to 1.5 cm of air. Proximal to the balloon, the thermistor (b) measures pulmonary artery temperatures. At a distance of 30 cm from the tip, the proximal port (c) is used to measure central venous pressures and to inject cold saline. All parts of the Swan-Ganz catheter must be thoroughly checked by flushing and inflation before it is inserted.

31

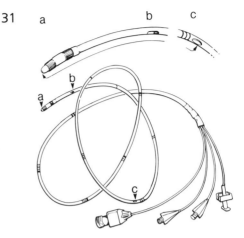

The anatomy of the area is again shown for reference.

32

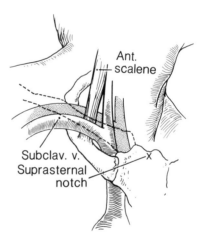

The area 2 to 3 cm below the middle of the clavicle is well infiltrated with 1% lidocaine and epinephrine. The cannulating needle is directed toward the sternal notch, and the subclavian vein is entered in the angle between the first rib and the clavicle.

33

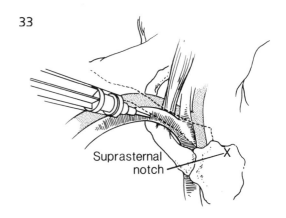

When the aspirating syringe confirms the free flow of blood, the floppy end of the guide wire is introduced and passed into the right atrium. The system must not be left open to the air for more than a fraction of a second because air embolism is such a serious complication; the needle must be covered with either a syringe or a finger or filled with a catheter or guide wire.

34

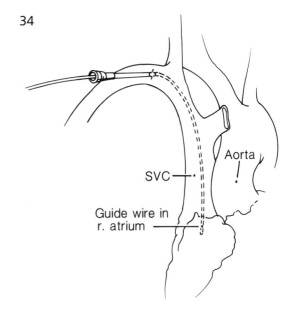

The needle is withdrawn from the guide wire. 35

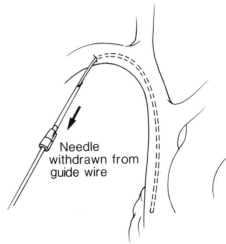

Needle
withdrawn from
guide wire

The dilator and introducer are threaded over the guide wire as a single unit. The dilator is advanced until the hub of the introducer is at the skin. 36

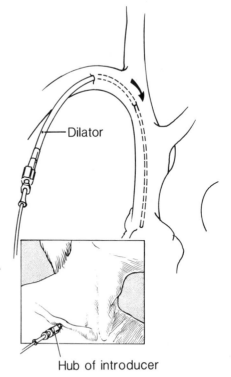

Dilator

Hub of introducer

The dilator and the guide wire are removed together, leaving the introducer in place. The lumen of the introducer is sealed with the finger to avoid the entrance of air and the loss of blood.

37

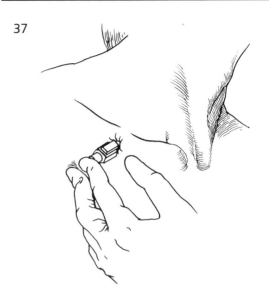

The Swan-Ganz catheter is threaded through the introducer. When the catheter is at the 20-cm mark, 1 ml of air is injected into the balloon. The catheter is attached to the pressure transducer and the pressure monitor, and the proximal port is filled with saline solution from a syringe that is left in place to prevent clotting and to allow for easy flushing.

38

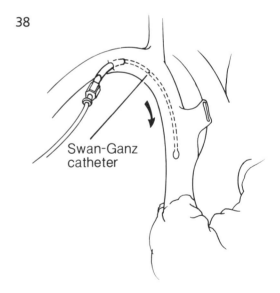

Swan-Ganz catheter

The catheter is advanced, allowing the balloon to guide it into the pulmonary artery. The progression of the tracings demonstrates the location of the tip of the balloon.

39

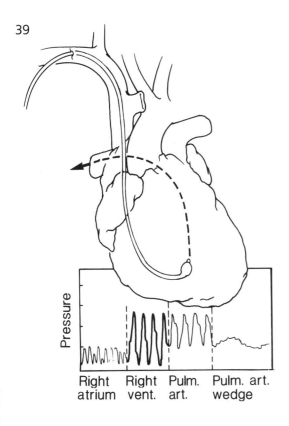

40

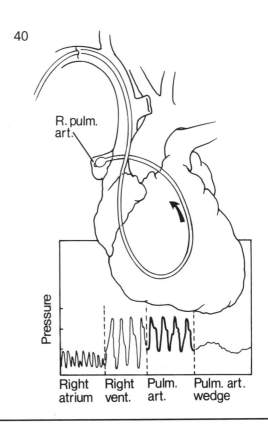

The change in tracing from the right ventricle to that of the pulmonary artery is demonstrated by the accented line. There is a change in the diastolic pressure as well as in the shape of the curve.

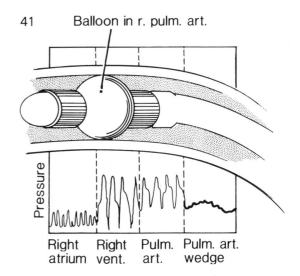

41   Balloon in r. pulm. art.

Right   Right   Pulm.   Pulm. art.
atrium vent.   art.   wedge

The catheter is advanced until the wedge tracing is seen. The balloon is collapsed. If the pulmonary artery tracing is restored and the wedge tracing is easily restored by introduction of less than 1.5 cm of air, the introducer is moved back over the catheter, and the catheter is sutured to the skin.

A roentgenogram of the chest is obtained as soon as the procedure is finished. The patient must be observed not only for the complications listed in the previous section but also for arrhythmias, thromboemboli, perforation of the pulmonary artery, and intracardiac knotting of the catheter.

Again, we emphasize that this is neither an office procedure nor one that is usually required of the family physician. It is included here because it is widely used and because every physician who is involved with the treatment of the seriously ill ought to be familiar with this technique of cardiac monitoring.

ARTERIAL PUNCTURE AND PLACEMENT OF ARTERIAL LINES

Access to arteries is only rarely needed in a family physician's office practice, but it is included here for reference should it be required in an emergency.

Arterial samples can be drawn most safely from the vessels of the wrist or the groin; if the vessels of the wrist are to be used, the collateral circulation of the hand must first be evaluated by an Allen test. The patient is asked to clench the fist, and both the radial and ulnar vessels are occluded by pressure against the bones of the wrist.

42

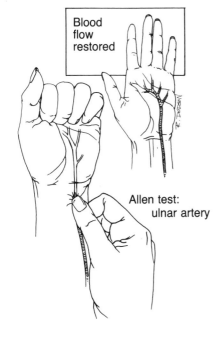

Blood flow restored

Allen test: ulnar artery

43

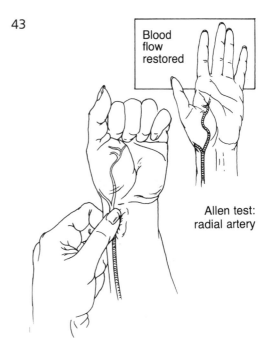

Blood flow restored

Allen test: radial artery

Each vessel should be tested individually. The hand should regain its color quickly when either artery is released. This is an important test. A significant number of individuals have only one or the other artery, and thrombosis of that vessel may lead to loss of digits or of the entire hand.

When no safe vessel is available in the wrist, the femoral artery can be used in both children and adults, but here also it is wise to rule out vascular pathology. The femoral vessel should *not be used* if there is any question about the blood supply of the limb or if the distal pulses are absent.

If an artery in the wrist is to be punctured, the skin is cleansed with an antibiotic solution, and the skin and the periarterial tissues are anesthetized with several milliliters of 1% lidocaine. Local anesthesia is not usually needed in punctures of the femoral artery.

44

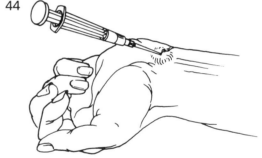

The artery is immobilized between two fingers, and a #20-gauge plastic-sheathed needle is aimed directly at it, positioned at an angle of 30 to 45 degrees. The needle is pushed through the artery and is then slowly withdrawn.

45

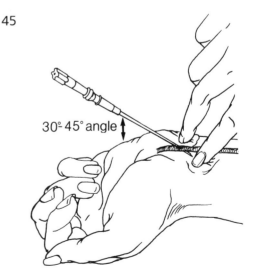

30°–45° angle

When arterial (bright red) blood is seen to spurt from the needle, the plastic sheath is advanced into the lumen of the artery, the needle is withdrawn, and the sample is collected in an appropriate container for analysis of the blood gases.

46

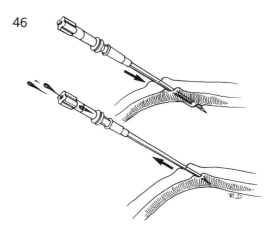

47

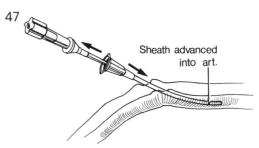

Sheath advanced into art.

If multiple arterial samples will be required, it is kinder to the patient to sew the cannula in place, fill it with a dilute heparin solution, and cap it until another sample is required.

48

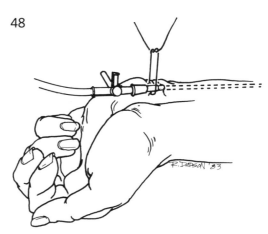

Arterial punctures can be complicated by thrombosis of the vasculature and by hematoma. Both of these complications must be watched for; in particular, the blood supply of the hand should be checked on a regular basis. If there is any question of ischemia, the catheter should be withdrawn and appropriate consultation requested without delay.

13 · *Thoracic Procedures and Emergencies*

WALTER J. PORIES, M.D.

Thoracic procedures that are appropriate for the office include thoracentesis, pleural biopsy, and treatment of broken ribs. We present several procedures that are also necessary for the care of thoracic emergencies because family physicians do see such cases, especially in civilian disasters and in remote areas.

ASSESSMENT OF PULMONARY FUNCTION

Before a patient is subjected to a thoracic procedure, he or she should be examined to assess pulmonary function and to determine whether the fluid is free or loculated within the pleural cavity. Pulmonary function can be adequately measured without any special instruments. Most important is the history; a record of smoking, asthma, previous pulmonary infections, and exposure to toxic or infectious agents may signal underlying disease. In addition, patients with chronic pulmonary disease frequently show evidence of weight loss, an increase in the dimensions of the chest cage, a greyish complexion, pursed lips with exhalation, and clubbing and, often, nicotine stains of the fingers. The accessory muscles of the neck frequently stand out as cords. Patients in acute pulmonary distress are usually cyanotic, anxious, and complaining of pain or tightness in the chest.

Assessment of the degree of ventilatory insufficiency can be accomplished by several easy maneuvers:

- Asking the patient to hold his or her breath as long as he or she can or to count as long as possible without taking a breath;

- Measuring the maximum distance at which the patient can extinguish a match by forceful exhalation *with the mouth open;*

- Determining how many steps a patient can climb before stopping because of shortness of breath;

- Measuring thoracic expansion and diaphragmatic movement with a cloth measuring tape at the level of the axillae; the difference between the measurement at maximum inspiration and at expiration represents the degree of thoracic expansion.

1

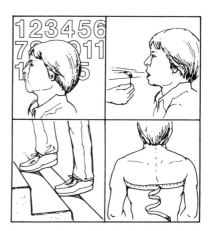

Relative expansion of the two sides of the chest can be compared by holding the patient's chest firmly, with the examiner's thumbs pointing at the scapulae. Variance in the movement of the thumbs reflects the variance in expansion between the two lungs.

2

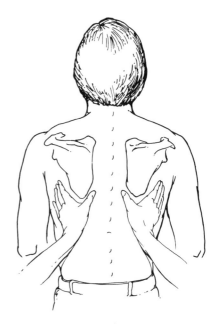

Percussion also can provide useful information about the location of the diaphragm, the degree of expansion of the underlying lung, and whether fluid is present and, if present, whether free or loculated. The diaphragm on the involved side is usually elevated, and its movement is limited. The degree of diaphragmatic motion can be determined by marking with a pen the lines where the percussion note changes from dull to resonant at maximum inspiration and expiration.

3a

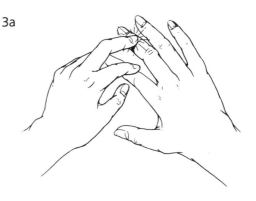

3b

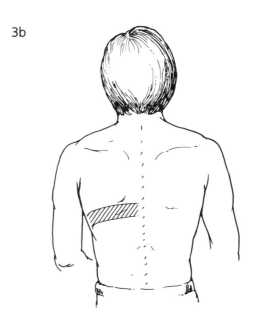

Free fluid shifts within the thoracic cavity with shift of position can be detected easily by movement of the area of dullness to percussion. The area of dullness is first identified with the patient in an upright position; its borders are marked out with a felt-tip or ballpoint pen. These boundaries are then compared with the area of

3c

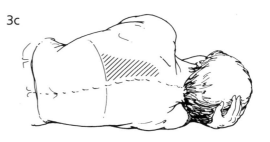

dullness in the new position. If there is no shift, either the fluid is loculated or the dullness is due to pulmonary disease or diaphragmatic paralysis.

Air can be distinguished from fluid because it is resonant rather than dull to percussion and because it can be detected best at the apex of the chest.

Because intrapleural fluid floats higher in the axillae than in the rest of the thorax, an axillary rise on percussion, often known as the S-line of Ellis, usually signals the presence of effusion, chyle, or blood.

4

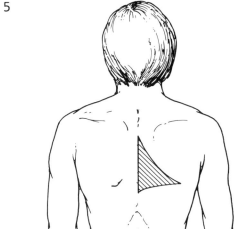

A triangular area of dullness usually indicates a collapsed lung.

5

Auscultation is also a useful and accurate tool for thoracic diagnosis, especially when X-ray facilities are not immediately available. The presence of normal breath sounds throughout both chest cavities usually is reliable evidence for absence of a pulmonary emergency. Generalized rales and wheezes suggest asthma or heart failure, localized rales usually signify pneumonia, and an accompanying wheeze suggests a stenotic lesion or tumor as the cause. If the lung is solid to percussion but transmits loud bronchial sounds, the bronchi are open, and the collapse is due to consolidation; if the breath sounds are not transmitted, the bronchus is closed, usually by a tumor.

THORACENTESIS

Thoracentesis—the aspiration of pleural fluid, either for diagnosis or for the relief of pleural compression—is not a difficult procedure if the fluid is free in the pleural cavity rather than loculated. Aspiration of loculated pockets is probably not an office procedure and, except in unusual circumstances, is best done under CAT scan or fluoroscopic control.

The procedure is best performed through the patient's back, with the subject straddling a chair. The position is comfortable, and the back of the chair lends stability. When the arms rest on the back of the chair, the scapulae are retracted out of the way, providing maximum access to the pleural spaces.

6

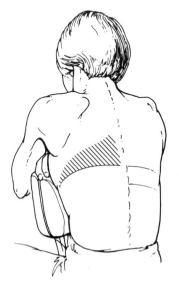

The site of the thoracentesis should be chosen carefully. The diaphragm is almost always higher on the involved side than on the normal side; a useful guide is to percuss out the level of the normal diaphragm and then insert the needle at least 4 in above that level in the involved side, just medial to the scapula.

Elaborate draping complicates the procedure and is unnecessary since there is little danger of contamination. We prefer merely to tape a towel under the selected site. The area is washed with a colored antiseptic solution such as Betadine.

7

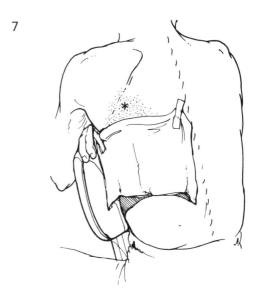

The equipment for thoracentesis includes two syringes (10 ml and 30 ml), two needles (#25 and #18), a three-way stopcock, and a #18 plastic-sheathed needle.

8

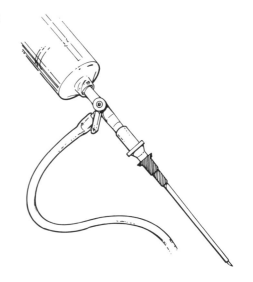

The skin, chest wall, and pleura are thoroughly infiltrated with about 10 ml of 1% lidocaine with epinephrine at the site of aspiration. Generous local anesthesia can make thoracentesis a painless procedure for the patient. A useful trick to ensure that the site will be productive is to advance the thin needle into the pleural cavity during injection of the anesthetic, for a test aspiration.

9

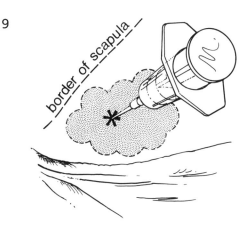

The large needle, its plastic sheath, and the three-way stopcock are then connected to the 30-ml syringe and a piece of IV tubing.

10a

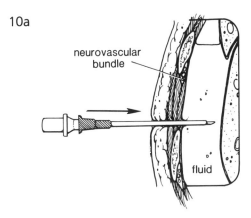

The needle is introduced into the chest so that it rides along the top of a rib to avoid damage to the neurovascular bundle of the interspace.

10b

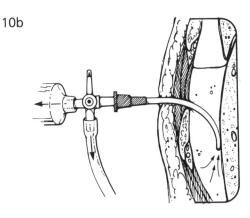

Entry of the needle into the pleural space is usually signaled by a pop and by the easy aspiration of fluid. At this point, the patient is asked to push down, grunt, or exhale, to avoid sucking air into the chest. The metal needle is withdrawn and the stopcock is quickly reattached to the cannula. The fluid can then be safely withdrawn through the soft cannula without fear of lacerating the lung. The fluid is aspirated into the syringe and discharged through the IV tubing, first into one or several test tubes in quantity sufficient for analysis, the rest being evacuated into a basin to be measured and discarded.

The fluid should be measured for volume, analyzed for specific gravity and protein content, and cultured for aerobic, anaerobic, and acid-fast bacteria and fungi. If malignancy is suspected, the fluid should be spun in a centrifuge and the sediment submitted for pathologic examination.

PLEURAL BIOPSY

When the etiology of the pleural effusion is in doubt, a pleural biopsy done at the time of thoracentesis may be helpful, particularly if the effusion has been present for some time or if the chest roentgenogram suggests pleural thickening.

The pleural biopsy is performed with an Abrams needle, a blunt, thick needle with a protected knife in its side. Because the biopsy is best done before much pleural fluid has been withdrawn, the following sequence is useful:

11

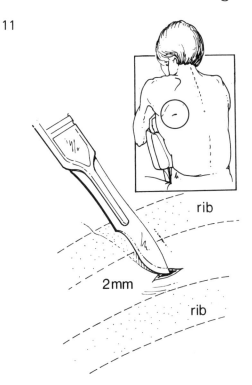

- Induction of local anesthesia

- Aspiration of sufficient fluid for cultures and pathologic examination

- Performance of pleural biopsy

- Evacuation of the remaining fluid

Insertion of the Abrams needle usually requires a small stab with a #11 or #15 blade, about 2 mm in length, to get through the skin. The needle is then pushed through into the pleural cavity so that it just grazes the top of the rib.

12a

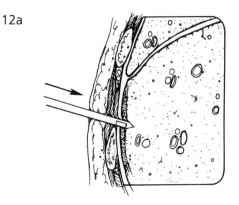

The inner cannula is retracted to expose the opening in the side of the needle and to capture tissue.

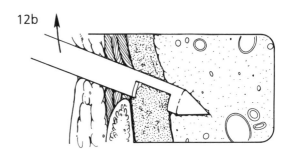

12b

The knife within the needle is advanced to obtain the biopsy, and the needle is withdrawn.

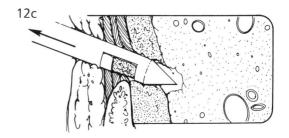

12c

A Band-Aid usually suffices as a dressing. Gross examination of the tissue is helpful in determining whether a useful biopsy has been obtained. If the specimen is red or yellow and soft, it usually includes only muscle or fat. Pathologic pleura is usually white or gray and firm or gritty in consistency.

DRAINAGE OF THE CHEST

Indications for prolonged drainage of the chest with a tube or needle include the presence of air, fluid, and blood within the pleural cavity. The most common condition (and often the most pressing emergency) is the pneumothorax.

Spontaneous pneumothorax is a common condition that can occur at all ages but is most common in young smokers and elderly patients with emphysema. The combination of acute lateral chest pain, dyspnea, and decreased breath sounds on the affected side is almost pathognomonic for the disease. The degree of pneumothorax that can be tolerated varies remarkably depending on the patient's pulmonary reserve; for example, it is common for a healthy athlete whose lung is totally collapsed on one side to deny dyspnea, while another patient with chronic pulmonary disease may be in dire straits from a pneumothorax of 10 to 20%.

Treatment is not necessary in all cases of spontaneous pneumothorax. A thin layer of air can be tolerated by most patients. Factors calling for earlier insertion of a chest tube include chronic pulmonary disease, increase of symptoms, and any obstacle to close observation of the patient. If possible, the presence and stability of the pneumothorax should be documented by serial chest roentgenograms, the first of which should include both inspiration and expiration films. Roentgenograms of the chest taken only on deep inspiration often fail to show a small pneumothorax because the air is stretched around expanded lung; in contrast, on expiration, the collection of air is larger in comparison to the lung compressed by exhalation and is thus more apparent.

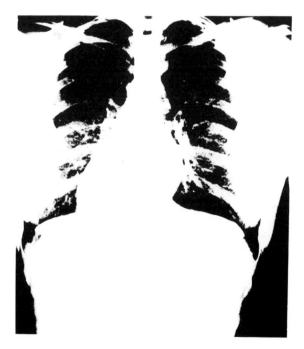

Inspiration

14

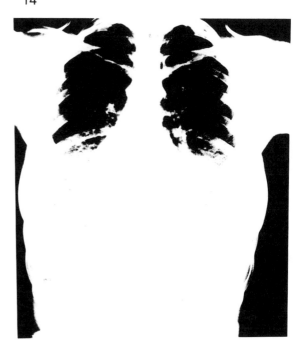

Expiration

There is a noteworthy rate of recurrence following pneumothorax; in general, 30% of all patients who have had one pneumothorax will have another; if a patient has had two, his or her chances of recurrence are at least 60%. Accordingly, serious consideration should be given to surgical pleurodesis if the patient has had two or more episodes and especially if a young patient is likely to be away from medical facilities during camping trips or similar endeavors. Surgical pleurodesis is not a big operation, carrying little more risk than the insertion of a chest tube. The procedure can be accomplished through a small incision in the armpit, by gently abrading the pleura with a sponge through the third intercostal space. The tube can usually be withdrawn and the patient discharged by the third day after surgery.

Pneumothorax may also be due to lacerations of the lung from fractured ribs, penetrating wounds, bronchial injuries, and other less common causes. In general, pneumothoraces caused by such conditions should be drained with a chest tube because they often remain unstable.

Fluid accumulations in the chest normally require chest tube drainage only if they are purulent or interfere with ventilation. Most pleural fluid will recede with resolution of the underlying cause; successful treatment of cardiac or renal failure or clearing of pneumonia will usually empty the pleural space as well. Particular caution is advised before insertion of a chest tube for a pleural effusion with malignancy. The chest wall is often lined with a friable carcinoma that bleeds readily, and insertion is occasionally impossible because of the reaccumulation of the effusion. Further, if the tube is left in longer than 10 days, the tumor may grow out of the tube site, presenting serious problems. If a tube is necessary for the comfort of patients with malignant effusions, it is often helpful to dry up the effusion, through installation of 1 gm of 5-fluorouracil or injection of a suspension of talc into the chest tube. This maneuver is successful in about half of such cases.

Unexplained pleural effusions are most commonly due to inflammatory processes under the diaphragm; causes such as pancreatitis, subphrenic abscess, or peritonitis must be ruled out in such cases.

Hemothorax, especially if associated with trauma, should uniformly be drained by a tube to avoid development of a constricting peel from the organizing clot and to allow measurement of the rate of blood loss. If after the original drainage blood continues to flow from the tube at a rate exceeding 100 ml per hour, thoracotomy will probably be necessary to arrest the bleeding.

In purulent effusions, the tube may often have to be left in place for weeks or even months, especially if there is an associated bronchopulmonary fistula. When the tube is required for more than 10 days, direct removal may not be possible if a track has developed that, if closed off by the pursestring suture, would become an abscess. Long-term tubes must therefore be allowed to extrude over several weeks (this procedure is discussed later).

Insertion of a Chest Tube

Insertion of a chest tube is a life-saving procedure that should be in the armamentarium of every family practitioner. The minimal equipment required should be available in the office for emergencies. The procedure is not difficult, but it can be terribly painful if the anesthetic is not liberally injected or if the incision is inadequate. The procedure can be dangerous if the tube is inserted too low. The diaphragm is usually elevated on the side with the pathology, and in such cases, one can easily skewer the spleen or liver. Such inadvertent intra-abdominal placement can usually be avoided by aspirating the pleural space with the needle and syringe used for the injection of the anesthetic agent; if fluid is not easily aspirated, the site is probably too low.

Another serious danger is associated with the use of trocars. These instruments are no longer widely used but are still present in some emergency rooms and therefore deserve special mention. The devices are thick metal cannulas measuring as much as 1 cm in diameter and consisting of a sharp inner steel core and a thin outer steel tube. The instrument is pushed into the chest with the help of the steel point, which is then withdrawn. The sheath guides the chest tube into the pleural space and is then removed around the tube, which is left in place. The instrument is dangerous because depth of placement may be hard to control, and one can easily plunge the trocar into the atrium or one of the great vessels of the chest.

Equipment needed for insertion of a chest tube includes the following items:

- 2 towels (1 to drape the patient, 1 to hold the instruments)

- 1% lidocaine with epinephrine (50 ml)

- 10-ml syringe

- #15 scalpel blade and handle

- Kelly clamp

- #28 chest tube (adequate for most problems). In children, a smaller tube may be required (#14–20); in patients with thick purulent effusions, a larger tube is sometimes helpful

- Two 3-0 monofilament sutures, such as Prolene, with cutting-edge needles

- Sponges

- 1-in tape

- Chest tube bottle and tubing (available as a sterile prepackaged set)

Suction is not usually needed in emergency situations. Most problems can be handled with the simple waterseal system described later.

In most cases, the best site of insertion is an incision through the mid-axillary line, just below the hairline, into the third intercostal space. The procedure is often facilitated for both patient and doctor by having the patient place the arm under the head and raising the back with a pillow or sandbag.

15

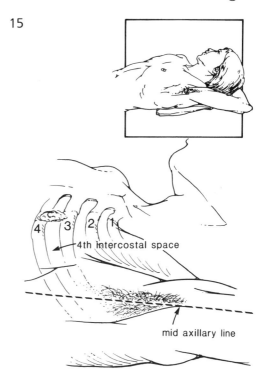

4th intercostal space

mid axillary line

The site is shaved, washed with an antiseptic, and *thoroughly* infiltrated with 20 to 30 ml of 1% lidocaine with epinephrine. The thoroughness of the anesthesia deserves emphasis, because without it the procedure is quite painful and the patient's (and indeed the staff's) co-operation is quickly lost.

A 3-cm incision is made through the skin just below the hairline, in the mid-axillary line, until fat is seen. At that site, axillary contents, lymph nodes, and large muscles of the chest wall are avoided. Only the fat lies between the skin and the intercostal muscles. The incision must be long enough to allow the clamp to introduce the catheter easily; much of the pain of this procedure is due to too-short incisions that require forcing of the clamp and the tube.

16

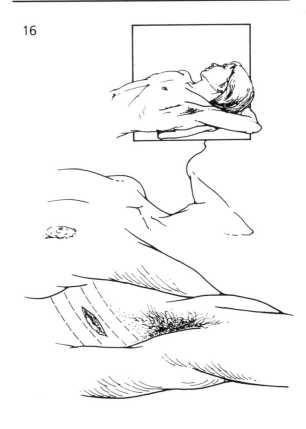

The fat is spread gently by the Kelly clamp. This will expose the intercostal muscles, which are then also punctured and spread by the clamp.

17

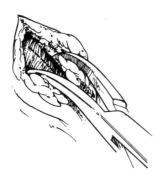

18

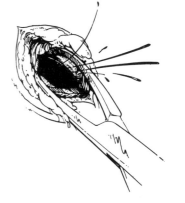

The burst of fluid or air usually encountered when the pleural space is entered may be surprising if it is not expected.

The chest tube is inserted between the jaws of the clamp and pushed into the pleural cavity at least 10 cm, or to the first black marker, so that all perforations in the cathether are within the pleural space. If difficulty is encountered, a finger may be inserted along the planned path of the catheter to determine whether the opening is large enough, whether the pleural space has indeed been entered, and whether there is pleurodesis or some other obstruction. The tube is then connected to the tubing that leads to the chest bottle and waterseal.

19

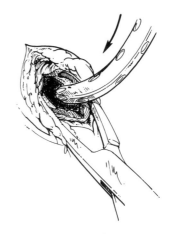

The tube is properly in place when the water level in the waterseal bottle rises and falls with each inspiration and expiration. This is an important sign; if the water level does not go up and down, the tube may be outside the pleural cavity, in the subcutaneous space or between the muscles.

20

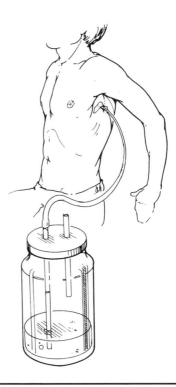

The chest tube is fastened by a suture approximating the skin edges around the tube to make an airtight seal. The suture is then wrapped about the tube several times to fasten it. This method, which resembles a Chinese finger trap, is more reliable and far easier than trying to tie the suture tightly around the tube.

21

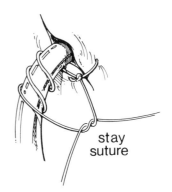

stay
suture

A second suture, a pursestring type, is then placed to ensure a seal when the chest tube is withdrawn.

22

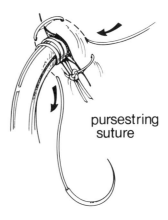

pursestring
suture

The pursestring suture is wrapped around a 2-×-2-in sponge to keep it from tangling, and the sponge is wrapped about the tube to serve as a dressing. The dressing is then taped in place.

23

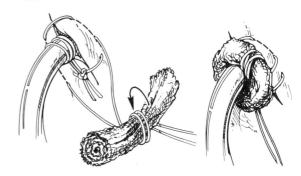

The tube is then attached to a chest bottle containing a thin layer of water covering the end of the drainage tube, to serve as a waterseal; thus, fluid and air can escape from the system but cannot flow back in. If wall or machine suction is available, it can be used at a setting of 20 to 30 cm of negative water pressure, but although it does empty the thorax more rapidly, it is usually not necessary. Waterseal alone normally does the trick.

Removal of a Chest Tube

The chest tube can be removed if the lung is fully expanded and if there has been no air leak for 24 hours, if the fluid output is less than 50 ml per day, or if the tube has been occluded for 24 hours. Chest roentgenograms should precede and follow removal of the chest tube.

The pursestring is unrolled from the dressing, tied with one knot, and held taut by the assistant. The suture holding the chest tube is then cut, and the patient is asked to take a deep breath and hold it (so that he won't gasp and suck air into the pleural space). The tube is withdrawn quickly with a jerk (stand aside—you can get splashed), and the pursestring is tied. A Band-Aid is applied. The pursestring suture can usually be cut and removed about 5 days later.

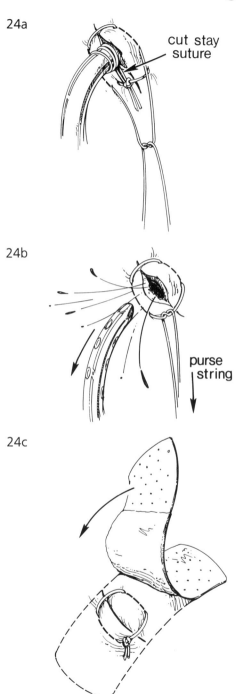

24a

cut stay suture

24b

purse string

24c

INSERTION OF A CLAGETT NEEDLE

Spontaneous pneumothorax in a good-risk patient can also be treated with a Clagett needle,
a curved stainless steel #14 needle with opposing perforations at its tip. The needle has
the advantage of being far easier to introduce
than a chest tube and leaves only a tiny scar.

25

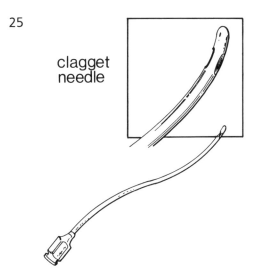

clagget
needle

A small wheal is made using 1% lidocaine with
epinephrine in the mid-axillary line just below
the hairline in the axilla.

26

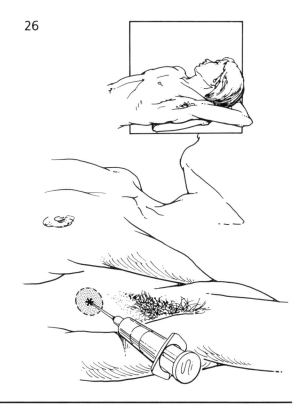

A 3- to 4-mm incision allows the introduction of the needle through the skin.

27

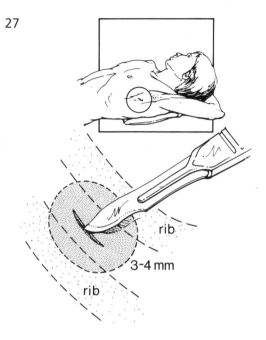

The needle is pushed into the chest through the intercostal space, and the curve of the needle is adjusted so that the needle comfortably follows the shape of the ribs.

28a

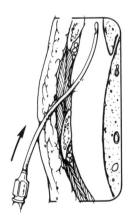

The needle is connected to an IV tubing's needle end; the other end of the IV tubing is cut off and taped to a glass or bottle of water so that the end of the tubing lies beneath the surface of the water and acts like a waterseal.

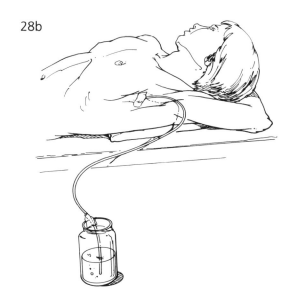

28b

One suture is usually needed to hold the needle in place, although tape can also be used. I have had excellent results with the Clagett needle and, in perhaps 80 to 90 cases, have seen it fail only once. The Clagett needle can usually be removed on the third day and the site covered with a small dressing for a day or two.

PERICARDIOCENTESIS

Pericardiocentesis—aspiration of fluid from the pericardial sac—is useful for sampling pericardial fluid for analysis or for emergency decompression of the tamponaded heart.

The patient lies supine upon a gurney or examining table, and the area around the xiphoid is cleansed with antiseptic. Anesthesia is usually not needed, but in anxious patients infiltration of the area with 1% lidocaine may be helpful.

29a

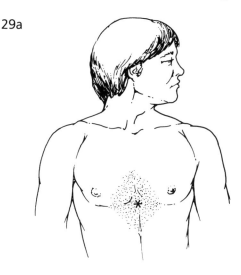

A #18 plastic-sheathed long needle attached to a three-way stopcock and a 30-ml syringe is introduced just below the xiphoid and aimed upward in the midline at an angle of about 45 degrees.

29b

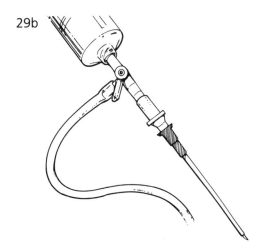

The pericardium is entered with a sharp pop; gentle aspiration should then yield either fluid or blood.

As soon as flow is established, the metal needle is withdrawn, leaving the plastic sheath within the pericardial cavity. This minimizes the possibility of injury to the coronary arteries and the ventricular wall. The remaining fluid is then removed and the needle withdrawn. A Band-Aid is applied.

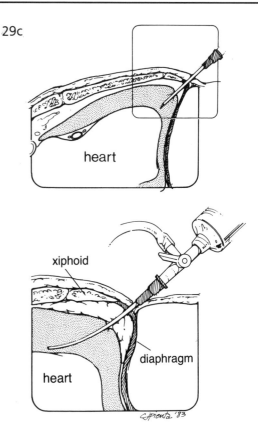

29c

heart

xiphoid

diaphragm

heart

The fluid is analyzed in a manner similar to that described for pleural fluid.

CARE OF THE SUCKING CHEST WOUND

Large penetrating injuries of the chest wall that communicate with the pleural space are called *sucking chest wounds* because air is sucked in and expelled with each breath. If the hole in the chest is about the size of the trachea or larger, it is easier for the air to enter through the wound than through the trachea, interfering with ventilation. Immediate treatment consists in sealing the hole with a cloth or sponge, whatever is at hand.

30

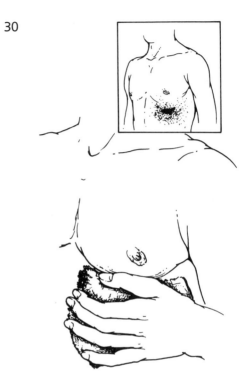

When the patient has been brought to an appropriate facility, ventilation is provided by an endotracheal tube, the chest is explored for other injuries, a chest tube is inserted, and the wound is thoroughly debrided and closed.

CARE OF RIB FRACTURES AND THE FLAIL CHEST

Rib fractures are common injuries, usually due to trauma, and are well tolerated although painful. If only one or two ribs are broken, if the underlying thoracic contents are not injured, and if the patient is in good health, reassurance and analgesia for 4 to 5 days usually suffice.

If a series of ribs is fractured—for example, ribs #3, 4, 5, 6, 7, and 8—or if a flail chest is present, patients may look deceptively well for the first few hours after injury and then become seriously ill. Initially, the patient may be able to splint the area successfully and remain well oxygenated, but within a few hours the splinted lung will become atelectatic, filling up with mucus or blood, and pneumonia may develop. As the patient tires, he or she is less able to splint, breathe effectively, or cough and becomes increasingly dyspneic and anoxic. Such patients require close observation and may benefit greatly from strapping, morphine, and antibiotics. If possible, they should be hospitalized for the first 24 to 48 hr to assess the severity of their injuries and their ability to cope with them. Baseline and follow-up electrocardiograms (EKGs) and cardiac enzyme studies should be performed to rule out a traumatic cardiac injury.

31

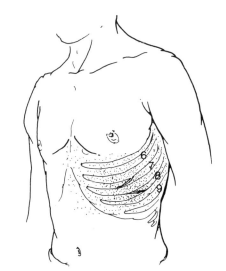

The location of the fractured ribs can provide important clues about potential underlying injuries. Fractures of the first and second ribs are often accompanied by injuries of the aortic arch or its major branches, fractures of the sternum suggest cardiac injuries, and fractures of the lower rib cage are frequently associated with injuries of the spleen or liver.

Strapping the Chest Wall

Strapping the chest wall can provide considerable comfort to the patient with fractured ribs. The possible danger of producing atelectasis to the underlying lung has been overemphasized; we have seen no ill effects from this procedure.

The area around the broken ribs is liberally painted with tincture of benzoin to protect the skin; at least two or three coats should be applied. Cloth tape 1-in wide is then applied in a herringbone interweaving pattern that extends over the two intact ribs above and below the fracture.

32

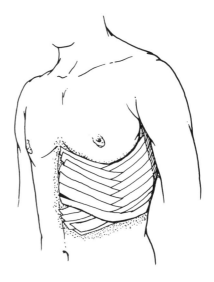

Intercostal Block

Some patients may benefit from an intercostal block. Somehow, the brief period of action of the local anesthetic often provides far longer relief than would be expected.

The block is administered to the involved ribs and two ribs above and below the fractures. The paravertebral area is cleansed with an antiseptic such as Betadine. In the midscapular line, or closer to the spine, if the ribs are fractured proximal to that area, a #20 needle with a syringe filled with 20 ml of 1% lidocaine is introduced under each rib into the hollow where the neurovascular bundle lies. About 4 to 5 ml are slowly injected into each site, producing a spotty area of anesthesia around the nipple.

Although many blocks last only a few hours, some patients may have relief for days or weeks. It is certainly worth a try in the patient who cannot be made comfortable with analgesic agents.

33

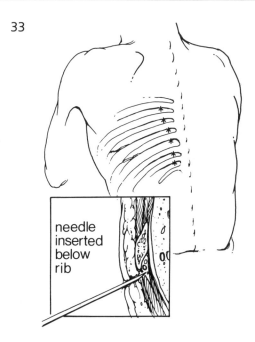

needle inserted below rib

Flail Chest

A flail occurs when several ribs are fractured in more than one place so that a segment of the chest wall flails, or moves ineffectively with respiration. The segment is sucked in during inspiration and blown out during expiration, moving the mediastinum back and forth. This produces an exchange of air from lung to lung (*Pendelluft,* or pendulum air, as the Germans term it) rather than ventilation through the trachea.

34a

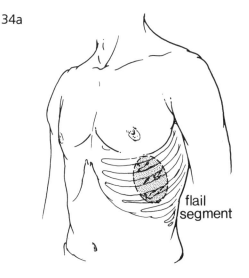

flail segment

34b

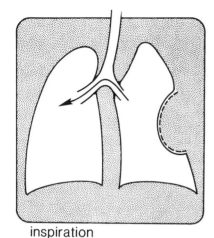

inspiration

34c

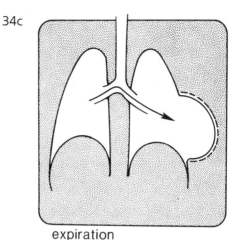

expiration

Emergency treatment of a flail chest calls for stabilizing the side by the simplest available means. In the field, this may mean simply placing a weight such as a stone against the flail, or, in the emergency room, a sandbag will do very well. This may immobilize the involved lung but at least it allows the rest of the lung to function.

A strong repeated caution is appropriate here: a patient with a flail chest may look deceivingly well during the initial hours after injury. At the least, such patients deserve hospitalization, and those with major flails will require long-term intubation and ventilatory support until the chest stabilizes.

14 · *Burns*

WALTER J. PORIES, M.D.

The skin is the body's largest organ and serves mainly as our protective envelope against the environment. It prevents the entry of microorganisms and toxins, regulates body heat and fluid balance, and functions as an organ of absorption, synthesis, and excretion. Burns involving relatively small areas of skin, as little as 5 to 10% of the total area, can have profound effects upon the body as a whole.

Unfortunately, burns are common, and family physicians are frequently faced with their care. This chapter emphasizes those aspects of burn care that are relevant to office practice: clinical evaluation of burns, office treatment of those burns that can be treated on an ambulatory basis, and emergency care and transport of burned patients who require hospital care.

EVALUATION OF THE BURNED PATIENT

Factors that influence the decisions about burn care include the following:

- Age of the patient

- Presence of other disease

- Cause, site, depth, and area of the burn

- Associated injuries

Age

Children under two years of age and adults over sixty tolerate burns far less well than patients between those ages. In both extreme age groups, the skin is far thinner than in patients in their middle years. In addition, infants have limited immunocompetence to fight infection, and the older adults often have associated diseases that increase mortality. Accordingly, patients in these two age groups should be admitted to the hospital if they have deep burns covering more than 5% of their skin surfaces or if the burns involve a critical site.

Presence of Other Diseases

Diabetes, chronic cardiac and pulmonary disease, malignancy, renal impairment, immunosuppression, and mental disease complicate the difficulties in burn treatment and increase the mortality. A major burn in a patient whose health is already compromised usually calls for hospitalization.

Cause of the Burn

The cause of the burn is an important determinant of care and outcome. Most burns are caused by thermal injury—from fire, explosions, steam, or contact with scalding liquids and hot objects. Of these, burns produced by contact are usually gravest because heat has been rapidly transferred to the tissues and the contact has frequently been prolonged. Sometimes, for example, with clothing made of nylon, the burning material adheres to and almost fuses with the skin; such prolonged contact at very high temperatures causes destruction of tissues that may extend into tendon and bone.

Contact burns may appear remarkably benign when first seen, even though they may be very deep. Scalds, in particular, are notorious for producing deep damage, even though the skin may retain a normal appearance; only close inspection will reveal the failure to blanch on contact and the characteristic pattern of thrombosed superficial veins. In contrast, although flash burns may have a frightening appearance, with black discoloration and bits of carbon, they can be surprisingly superficial. Thus, the cause of the burn is an important clue to the degree of tissue damage.

Chemical and electrical burns are particularly hazardous. Chemical burns may continue to damage tissues long after the initial contact, especially if the burning agent is one that cannot be readily removed, such as phosphorus. Electrical burns can produce extensive tissue damage that may also be inapparent; the so-called wounds of entry and exit can be deceptively small and yet conceal coagulation throughout the full thickness of a limb.

Site of the Burn

Burns of the face, perineum, and hands are most likely to be associated with serious complications. Burns of the face may involve the eyes and ears and often herald burns of the airway and inhalation injuries to the lungs. Perineal burns are difficult to keep clean and are therefore usually complicated by infection and poor healing. Burns of the hands are likely to be deep, especially on the thin-skinned dorsal surface; scarring can all too readily limit function in the hands permanently.

Depth of the Burn

The depth of the burn is described as first, second, or third degree. *First-degree burns* involve only the epidermis and are usually caused by brief scalding or by excessive exposure to the sun. Tissue damage is slight, and the skin is usually bright red, with mild edema; pain is the major symptom. Systemic symptoms, if any, are usually mild and may include nausea, fever, and generalized weakness. Symptoms usually resolve within 48 hr, and healing, often associated with peeling, is usually complete within a week.

Second-degree burns extend beyond the epidermis into the dermis and may vary from superficial, which may be only slightly deeper than first degree, to deep, which may involve the destruction of all but a few deep epidermal remnants. Superficial second-degree burns usually show blistering, little loss of sensation, and considerable pain; deep burns are often insensitive and surprisingly painless.

The rate of healing depends on the degree of destruction. Superficial burns are resurfaced quickly from the rete pegs and epidermal appendages and usually heal with minimal scarring in less than two weeks. Deep burns may take months to heal because all of the epithelium has to be regenerated from a few remaining islands. The dermis does not regenerate and is replaced by a thick scar that causes immobility and contractures of the underlying structures. Because the new epithelium is usually only a thin sheet without the anchoring properties of the rete pegs, it is easily wiped off and lost with simple injuries, bringing about recurrent ulceration, which, in time, may lead to a squamous carcinoma, or so-called Marjolin's ulcer.

Third-degree burns are those burns that destroy the full thickness of the epidermis, extending deeply into the dermis and often into the deeper tissues. These burns often have the appearance

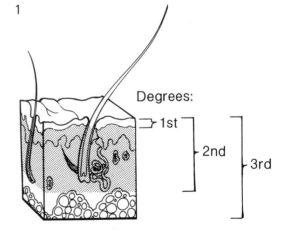

1

Degrees:

of tanned leather, and a network of thrombosed veins is often visible under the anesthetic surface.

It is often difficult to distinguish between second- and third-degree burns, especially when the level of the second-degree burns is deep. If large enough—covering more than 5% of the body surface—both can produce profound metabolic abnormalities.

Third-degree burns heal even less well than deep second-degree burns. As no nests of epithelium remain, all of the coverage has to originate from the perimeter of the burn. Further, the destruction of the dermis and its replacement by scar deprive the epithelium of cushion and adequate nutrition. Avoidance of infection of the burn is therefore essential because resultant destruction of the remaining dermis and nests of epithelium will change a second-degree burn that can heal into one of third degree that may not.

The chief aims in local burn care are thus twofold: support of the healing process and prevention of destruction of the remaining nests of epithelium by infection.

Area of the Burn

The surface area of the burn is one of the main determinants of survival. The size of the burn is usually expressed as a percentage of body area and is best estimated with the so-called rule of nines. There is a considerable difference between the surface areas in children and in adults.

In general, complete healing is not possible when a deep burn is larger than the palm of the patient's hand. Lesions of this size usually require skin grafting.

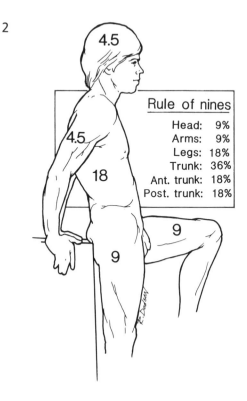

Rule of nines

Head:	9%
Arms:	9%
Legs:	18%
Trunk:	36%
Ant. trunk:	18%
Post. trunk:	18%

Associated Injuries

Patients frequently sustain other injuries when they are burned, especially if they are hurt during such events as industrial accidents or explosions or in wartime. Associated injuries vastly complicate the care of a burn and are often overlooked. Fractures, brain injuries, inhalation burns, compression injuries of the abdomen, and easily missed missile entry and exit wounds are common companions of burns.

In summary, the following categorization of burn severity developed by the American Burn Association is a most helpful guide to the evaluation of the burned patient.

3

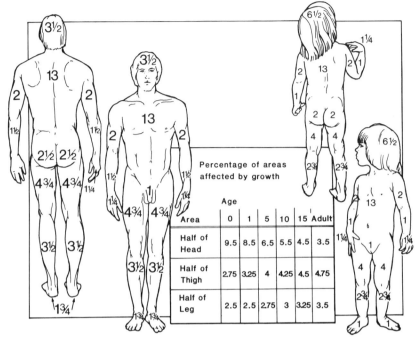

Percentage of areas affected by growth						
Age						
Area	0	1	5	10	15	Adult
Half of Head	9.5	8.5	6.5	5.5	4.5	3.5
Half of Thigh	2.75	3.25	4	4.25	4.5	4.75
Half of Leg	2.5	2.5	2.75	3	3.25	3.5

Summary of the American Burn Association Categorization of Burn Severity*

Major Burn Injury
Second-degree burns > 25% of body surface area in adults
Second-degree burns > 20% of body surface area in children
Third-degree burns > 10% of body surface area
Most burns involving hands, face, eyes, ears, feet, or perineum
Most patients with the following: inhalation injury; electrical injury; burn injury complicated by other trauma
Poor-risk patients with burns

Moderate, Uncomplicated Burn Injury
Second-degree burns of 15 to 25% of body surface area in adults
Second-degree burns of 10 to 20% of body surface area in children
Third-degree burns of < 10% of body surface area

Minor Burn Injury
Second-degree burns < 15% of body surface area in adults
Second-degree burns < 10% of body surface area in children
Third-degree burns < 2% of body surface area

*Handbook of Surgery, 7th Edition, ed. Theodore R. Schrock, M.D. Greenbrae, CA: Jones Medical Publications, 1982, p. 18.

TREATMENT

Triage

One of the crucial decisions in the care of the burn patient is whether to treat the patient as an outpatient or to admit him or her to the hospital. It is easy to underestimate the severity of burns and to minimize the additive effects of preexisting disease and associated additional injuries. Further, in many patients, the burn is not really accidental, as it may appear; burns are frequently the result of attempted homicidal or suicidal acts, and such patients are often severely disturbed. If there is doubt, it is better to admit the patient to a hospital for initial observation.

The preceding American Burn Association categorization of burns is a useful guide. In general, patients who sustain burns listed as minor can be treated in the office and at home; those with severer injuries should be referred to a hospital.

Emergency Treatment of Serious Burns

Remarkably little needs to be done for most patients with severe burns to prepare them for transport to a hospital, even if the facility is an hour away. If the patient arrives within half an hour after the burn, the injured areas should be treated as soon as possible with cold compresses to minimize thermal damage. An airway and ventilatory support must be secured if there is an indication of inhalation injury or poisoning by carbon monoxide or other fumes. Open wounds should be dressed; fractures should be splinted. If there is indication of a spinal cord injury, the usual steps of preventing further neurologic damage need to be followed.

If it can be done readily, an IV should be started and lactated Ringer's solution administered at a rate of about 100 ml/hr during transport. If the tissues are too badly burned, however, it is usually best to proceed with transport so that hospital personnel can do the cutdown. The procedure is often difficult and time consuming, and there is rarely a rush to administer the fluids unless associated injuries are severe enough to cause hypovolemia.

Dressing care of the major burn is best deferred until the patient gets to the hospital. During transport, the patient can be covered with clean cloths or sheets, injuries can be dressed minimally in the usual manner, and fractures should be splinted. This approach saves time and permits the receiving physicians to assess the extent and depth of the burn themselves. If debridement or cleansing of the burn must be done, it can be performed in the hospital under better conditions and with the patient under anesthesia.

It is particularly important to secure as good a medical history as possible immediately after the burn because these patients may only be lucid for one to a few hours. Tetanus prophylaxis should be initiated in all cases. A Foley catheter should be placed and a careful record of intake and output with hourly measurements begun. The use of prophylactic antibiotics is usually discouraged, although some physicians still favor the use of penicillin for three days to prevent early infection with streptococcus.

Outpatient Care of Minor Burns

4

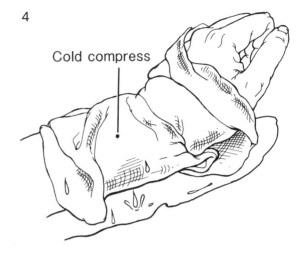

Cold compress

The best immediate emergency treatment of any burn is to wash or immerse the part in cold water to reduce the temperature of the tissues as quickly as possible. There is ample evidence that prompt cooling can reduce a potential deep second-degree burn to only superficial damage. A friend of one of the authors watched with horror as a waitress accidentally spilled a pot of boiling water over his young son, then admired her presence of mind as she rapidly scooped up the glasses of ice water from the table and poured these over the child. The infant sustained no serious burn. Cooling is, of course, most effective if it is done immediately, but it can still be of help when the patient is first seen. Tissues hold heat for a long time; even a half hour after the injury there may still be enough heat in the tissues to continue producing damage. In addition, the application of cold compresses is soothing and comforting to the anxious patient and the family. Accordingly, it is good practice to treat the patient immediately with cold applications upon arrival in the office or the emergency room, leaving these in place for about a half hour.

The burned area should then be cleaned gently with soap and water or a mild antiseptic such as Betadine. Grease, oil, dirt, and other foreign matter should be flushed or wiped away as delicately as possible. If it hurts, it's not being done right.

5

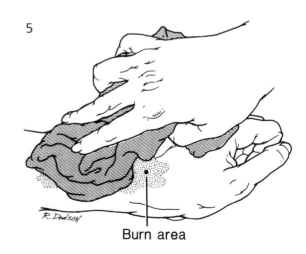

Burn area

A careful record should be made of the extent and suspected depth of the burn; a drawing, indicating the distribution of discoloration, change in sensation, blistering, and other surface changes, is particularly useful. In addition, the vascular supply and function of the part should be carefully tested and recorded. Fractures, other deep injuries, and foreign bodies need to be sought and treated. If a chemical burn is suspected, lavage should be copious, and information should be sought from the Poison Control Center about appropriate local antidotes and possible systemic effects.

6

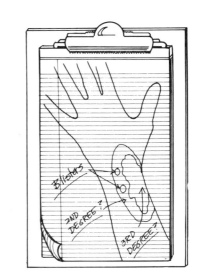

Debridement should be gentle and minimal. Although there is controversy about the best treatment of blisters, the authors prefer to leave them alone unless they are particularly bothersome to the patient. In such cases, we make a small puncture wound at the edge of the blister with a needle and allow the fluid to escape, thus allowing the elevated epidermis to serve as a temporary cover until the new epidermis resurfaces the area. We observe that patients treated in this manner have considerably less pain than when the blister is uncovered.

7

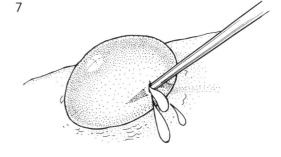

Minor burns are best dressed with a single layer of fine-mesh gauze impregnated with a mild antiseptic ointment or cream; Furacin or Betadine gauze works well for superficial burns and is supplied in a readily available form in sterile envelopes. For deeper burns, we prefer to use Silvadene ointment to minimize infection. The salve soothes the skin and almost immediately reduces the pain; the antiseptic may be helpful in minimizing infection. The fine mesh is then

8

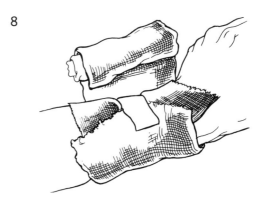

covered with a bulky absorbent dressing made of Kling, abdominal pads, or a similar product. The dressing can be left undisturbed for four to five days if the patient remains well. The gauze can then be soaked off with water to avoid tearing the newly healing tissues; frequently the area is almost healed and will need only a dry dressing. If there are still granulations, as in a medium-level-deep second-degree burn, the same kind of dressing is reapplied every few days until healing is complete.

A new type of dressing, OP-Site, has proven to be excellent for the treatment of minor burns. The material, which resembles thin cellophane, serves as an artificial epidermis. It controls pain almost instantaneously and seems to encourage healing as well as any approach we have seen. This type of dressing is left undisturbed until healing is complete, at which time it automatically falls off.

9

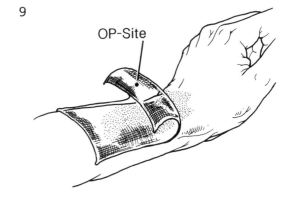

OP-Site

Prophylaxis against tetanus should always be instituted. Antibiotics are usually not necessary but can be given for short periods if there is considerable soiling or if the patient's resistance is in doubt.

The function of the burned part must be maintained. The skin should be kept supple with emollients such as Crisco or cocoa butter, and joints should be kept functional and mobile with appropriate splinting and aggressive physiotherapy.

If a burn takes longer than three weeks to heal, or if the granulating surface exceeds 5×5 cm, consideration should be given to skin grafting. It will not only shorten the period of recovery but also will produce a more functional and cosmetic cover and diminish contracture. This is particularly true of the face and hands.

Patients with burns should be warned about the signs of infection and instructed to notify the physician if they develop fever, unusual discomfort, edema of the limb, or lymphadenitis. Streptococcus is most commonly the responsible organism, and penicillin will usually clear the erysipelas quickly.

Many patients with burns are emotionally ill or come from broken homes or disturbed family situations. The physician should be certain that there is an adequate support system before assuming that the burn can be cared for at home. When doubt exists, it is often safer to admit the patient to the hospital for a day or so until the situation can be thoroughly investigated.

III · *Special Problems*

15 · *Surgical Procedures in Ophthalmology*

STEVEN M. WHITE, M.D.

Several surgical conditions of the eye can be handled safely in the family physician's office. These include the removal of a corneal foreign body and the treatment of an acute chalazion and hordeolum. Test the vision and examine the eye carefully by gross inspection and with the ophthalmoscope before undertaking any one of these procedures.

CORNEAL FOREIGN BODY REMOVAL

A superficially embedded corneal foreign body can usually be removed with the use of a sharp, sterile hypodermic needle and one of the topical anesthetic agents, such as 1/2% tetracaine. If the corneal foreign body has been present for several days and there is an infiltrative reaction seen in the cornea under close inspection, the patient should be referred to an ophthalmologist. If there is no reaction in the surrounding cornea and the foreign body is superficially embedded, it usually can be removed without difficulty. Underlying staining of the corneal stroma is a fairly common occurrence following removal of the foreign body, especially if the foreign body contains iron. If the staining is minimal and is not over the central pupillary zone, the patient can be treated with prophylactic antibiotic drops. A combination of neomycin, polymyxin, and bacitracin drops, such as Neosporin, is best instilled into the eye at a rate of one drop every two waking hours for two or three days, or until the eye is asymptomatic.

If foreign body sensation is noticeable by the following day, the patient should be referred to an ophthalmologist.

1a

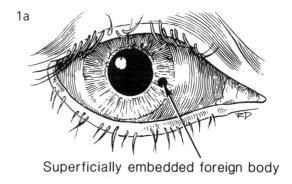

Superficially embedded foreign body

1b

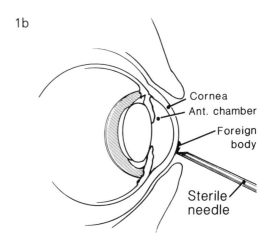

Cornea
Ant. chamber
Foreign body
Sterile needle

If the corneal foreign body is in the central pupillary zone, the patient should also be referred to an ophthalmologist. The removal of a corneal foreign body should be attempted only when the room is lighted adequately, the patient is cooperative, and the physician is wearing a pair of magnifying binocular loupes. Steroid drops should never be used in the presence of any corneal epithelial defect.

Figure 1a and b shows a fairly large superficially embedded corneal foreign body and its removal with a hypodermic needle.

ACUTE CHALAZION AND HORDEOLUM

A hordeolum is an infection of a sebaceous appendage of the lash follicle and usually points on the lid border. During the acute stage, it is frequently quite painful, produces a focal cellulitis, and is best treated with moist, warm compresses. Systemic antibiotics are rarely necessary. The lesion will usually open and drain within two or three days. If the lesion points and fails to drain, and there is a focal abscess visible underneath the skin, a superficial stab incision with a #11 Bard-Parker blade will drain the lesion and afford the patient relief.

2a

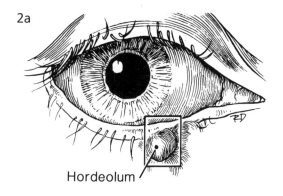

Hordeolum

2b

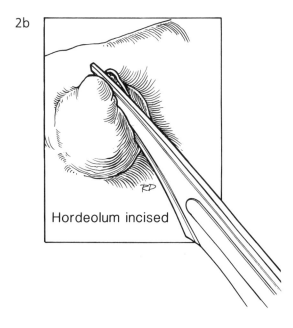

Hordeolum incised

A chalazion is an obstruction of the meibomian gland of the tarsal cartilage of the upper or lower lid, usually associated with some mild inflammatory reaction. Occasionally, in the presence of an acute infection, an abscess can occur. If an abscess can be seen pointing within the chalazion, incision and drainage will again afford the patient relief. Often a subacute chalazion points with granulomatous tissue, and the dome of the lesion appears yellow rather than white. Attempts at drainage of such a chalazion will be nonproductive. The general treatment of chalazion consists of moist, hot compresses; if the lesion fails to resolve within two or three weeks, the patient should be referred to an ophthalmologist.

3a Chalazion with abcess pointing beneath skin

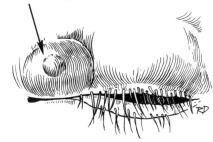

3b Abcess incised

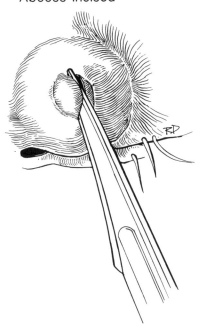

16 · *Otolaryngologic Procedures*

PAUL S. CAMNITZ, M.D.

EARS

Myringotomy

Myringotomies are most often done for chronic serous otitis and are usually performed prior to placement of a ventilation tube. In both instances, the patient should be referred to an otolaryngologist. However, myringotomies may occasionally be done by a family physician for diagnostic purposes or relief of pain.

Otitis media will sometimes be associated with or precede severer infections. Partially treated otitis sometimes accompanies pneumonia, meningitis, and fever of unknown origin. In such cases, the ear problem does, otitis is but a grave

problem and there is time for the fluid to be removed, prepared with a Gram's stain, and cultured to indicate the appropriate therapy.

In infants, no anesthesia is used. The child is wrapped in a sheet or placed in a papoose-type restrainer. Myringocentesis is then performed by means of a tuberculin syringe and a 1-1/2-in 25-gauge needle, with the aid of an operating head otoscope. Sedation with a so-called cardiac cocktail is frequently helpful (meperidine hydrochloride, 25 mg/cc; Phenergan, 6.25 mg/cc; and chlorpromazine hydrochloride, 6.25 mg/cc, given at a dosage of 1 cc/10 kg of body weight IM, up to 2 cc 30 to 45 min before the procedure). Myringocentesis should always be by way of the inferior portions of the tympanic membrane, preferably in the anterior-inferior quadrant, where there are no vulnerable underlying middle-ear structures.

A definite indication for myringotomy is acute otitis media with a bulging tympanic membrane, indicating increased middle-ear pressure, accompanied by intractable pain. Choice of anesthesia depends on the age and psychologic make-up of the patient. Although the ear canal in cooperative adults can be injected with lidocaine, proceeding without any anesthesia is more comfortable if the patient will tolerate it. The myringotomy incision is usually accomplished with only minimal discomfort in a tympanic membrane under constant pressure and tension from the otitis. In like manner, local anesthesia is best avoided in infants who can be immobilized.

Conversely, one should not hesitate to use general anesthesia for the fearful child or adult who cannot be safely restrained. The most experienced ear surgeon would have difficulty avoiding injury to the delicate middle-ear structures in an uncooperative child.

Myringotomy requires the patient to be supine with the head turned so that the affected ear is pointing upward; this helps prevent withdrawal of the tympanic membrane and allows for easy, passive restraint of the head. An otoscope with an operating head is far superior to the windowed otoscopes because it allows the surgeon to work with adequate magnification.

The myringotomy knife is introduced through the speculum, care being exercised to avoid touching the walls of the ear canal. Contact with the canal wall will cause discomfort, undermining the patient's efforts to remain immobile, and can cause troublesome bleeding, obscuring the surgeon's view.

The myringotomy should be done under direct vision in the posterior-inferior quadrant of the pars tensa. Because the tympanic membrane is usually thickened by the infectious process, considerable pressure may be required for a through-and-through incision. Pain relief will be immediate.

1

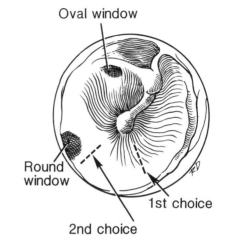

Foreign Body Removal

Foreign bodies that are easily seen without an otoscope can be removed with forceps. More frequently a foreign body (insects, cotton, beads, pencil erasers, paper) is pushed inward toward the isthmus of the ear canal (the point where the bony canal meets the cartilaginous canal). At this point, the ear canal is not distensible, and manipulation is painful because of tight adherence of the skin, periosteum, and bone. Initial attempts to remove the foreign body should be by means of gentle warm-water irrigation. The pinna is pulled upward and back, thereby aligning the cartilaginous and bony canals. If this maneuver does not dislodge the object, attempts can be made to withdraw the foreign body through an otoscope using a small, blunt, right-angle hook or cup forceps. In adults, if such efforts become painful, local anesthesia can be achieved by injecting the ear canal with 1% lidocaine with epinephrine. In children this is usually not possible, and general anesthesia is an absolute requirement.

2

Points where bony canal meets cartilaginous canal

Special mention should be made of insects. Patients commonly complain of a crawling sensation in the ear. It may be all but impossible to remove a live insect from the patient's external canal in the office. An easy way to deal with the problem is to instill 3 to 4 cc of ether into the ear canal and to withdraw it 2 to 3 min later. Make sure to examine the canal closely afterward to be sure that the entire creature has been removed.

Cerumen impactions are another special case. Unless the patient has used a makeshift curette (bobby pin, Q-tip, etc.), there is usually no trauma to the canal or inflammation. One should first try the standard techniques of suction, ear wax curettes, and irrigation, the latter by means of a large syringe and body-temperature water. If the water is not at body temperature, the patient will become profoundly dizzy. One should take special care to avoid total occlusion of the ear canal by the tip of the syringe; there must be a constant escape route for any water put into the canal. Impacted cerumen can be loosened by instilling a 1:1 mixture of hydrogen peroxide and glycerin in the ear canal and leaving it in place for 15 to 20 min. Recalcitrant patients, without accompanying infection, can be directed to use any one of the commercially prepared anticerumen ear drops for 7 to 10 days, after which they should return for follow-up and removal.

3a

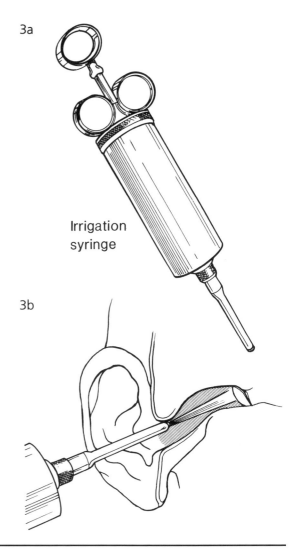

Irrigation syringe

3b

NOSE

Epistaxis

Nasal hemorrhage most often occurs between the ages of 10 and 13; its incidence then decreases until middle age, when it rises again to a lower peak. Epistaxis can be life threatening; it is therefore important for family practitioners to know the proper treatment. The family practitioner should be able to arrest and treat simple anterior nosebleeds as well as to control serious nasal hemorrhage until definitive therapy can be carried out.

The arterial supply of the nose comes from both the external and internal carotid systems. The most common site of bleeding is the anterior nasal septum, in an area of anastomoses between these two systems. This area, called Kisselbach's plexus, is where the septal branch of the superior labial artery, the greater palatine artery, the septal sphenopalatine artery (all in the external carotid system), and the anterior ethmoidal artery (internal carotid system) conjoin.

4

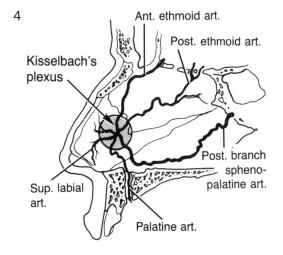

There are several reasons why the nose is a frequent site of bleeding. The mucosa over Kisselbach's plexus is subject to constant drying by air. Any defect of the mucous barrier or the ciliated mucosal lining (as in viral infection or allergic rhinitis) can cause erosion over the vessels, which have very little surface protection. The septal skeleton is covered first by perichondrium or periosteum and then by the vascular tissue layer. Superficial to these layers is a very delicate mucosa. Absence of cushioning and of surrounding muscle makes these vessels less likely to contract than other vessels; they are therefore less likely to stop bleeding spontaneously.

One should approach the treatment of epistaxis stepwise. More than 90% of cases can be controlled by simple nasal compression. This should be maintained for 10 min. If this does not stop the bleeding, the physician should then gown both him- or herself and the patient. Suction should be available. An angulated sucker tip is helpful; good light source is imperative; cocaine, either 4 or 10%, is placed on cotton pledgets that are inserted into the nose and left in place for 1 min. If cocaine is not available, a cotton ball saturated with 1:1,000 epinephrine can be substituted and placed in the nose for 2 min.

5

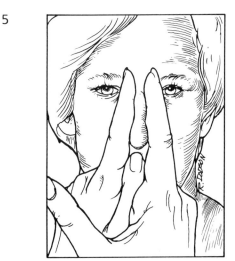

Any bleeding points can be cauterized with silver nitrate sticks, held on the bleeding point for 20 to 25 sec. Perforation is unlikely because this cauterization is very superficial. If the bleeding point lies in Kisselbach's triangle, one should make concentric circles inward toward the bleeding point, the outer circle being approximately 1 cm in diameter. Any excess silver nitrate should be removed. Electrocoagulation is occasionally necessary, particularly for lateral-wall defects. Anesthesia is obviously necessary and can be accomplished with cocaine, lidocaine, or both.

6

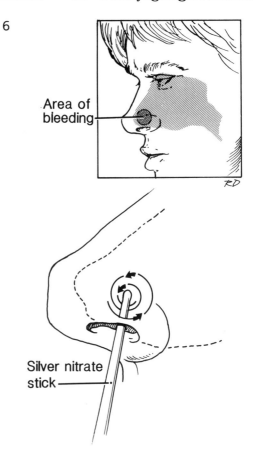

Area of bleeding

Silver nitrate stick

If cauterization stops the bleeding, a wet Gelfoam packing in the nose will usually maintain hemostasis, protecting the cauterized area from the drying effects of inspired air.

Occasionally the nose will continue to bleed despite the measures mentioned, in which case 1/2-in ribbon gauze, impregnated with either Vaseline or Neosporin, is the standard packing material to use. By means of bayonet forceps, the ribbon is first passed along the floor of the nose, then built up in successive loops from the floor upward, to exert an even pressure on the whole nasal mucosa. The pack is left in place for 48 to 72 hr, and the patient is allowed to go home. Patients with nasal packing should have prophylactic antibiotic coverage because the packing blocks the ostia to the paranasal sinuses, increasing the risk for acute sinusitis.

If the nasal hemorrhage continues, or if the patient has a posterior bleeding point, some type of posterior pack is necessary. Several commercially available posterior nasal balloons are adequate for short-term therapy; these are usually double- or triple-lumen catheters with inflatable balloons for tamponade. If such devices are not available, a Foley catheter can be placed in the nasopharynx via the nose, then filled with air or saline solution and wedged back into the posterior choana for tamponade of the posterior bleeding point. An anterior pack is then placed in front of this. These methods are temporary.

A more permanent posterior pack can be fashioned of 2-×-2-inch gauze packs; usually five to eight pieces are sutured together at two diagonal corners. The sutures are left long for further use. A catheter is inserted through the nose and pulled out through the mouth. The pack is tied to the catheter and then brought back through the nose and wedged into the choana, by maintaining constant pressure on the suture coming through the nose while using the opposite-hand index finger to direct the pack around the palate and into the nasopharynx.

7

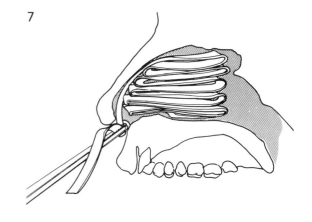

8a

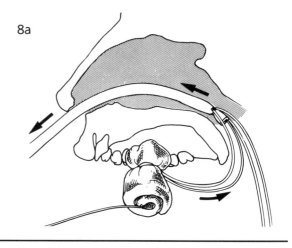

8b

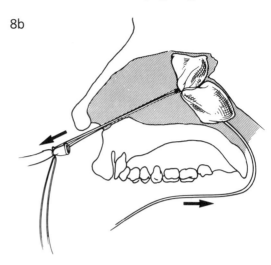

8c

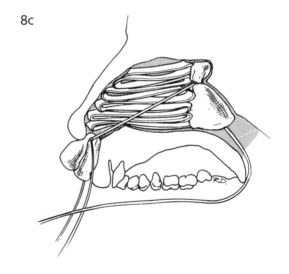

An anterior pack is then inserted, and the two sutures on the corners of the posterior pack are tied together over a dental roll. The anterior pack is thus held in place by "bookending" between the posterior pack in back and the dental roll in front. This method of treatment must be carried out on both sides. The suture from the diagonal corners of the pack is brought out through the mouth and taped to the cheek to facilitate future removal.

The pack is left in place for 72 hr, during which time the patient is hospitalized. Antibiotics are again a must. One should carefully monitor the respiratory status of patients with nasal packs, as nasal packs are known to cause a reflex drop in pO_2.

If packing does not stop the bleeding, the patient should be referred for a more extensive surgical procedure such as ligation of the anterior and posterior ethmoidal arteries and either the ipsilateral internal maxillary artery or the external carotid artery. This is a highly successful procedure and has a low morbidity. Once the patient's bleeding has been stabilized, the physician must seek the cause of the hemorrhage.

Foreign Body Removal

Foreign bodies in the nose are usually seen in children under five years old. The child routinely denies the presence of any foreign body, probably from a combination of embarrassment and fear of punishment. The usual clinical picture is that of unilateral foul-smelling nasal discharge that has gone on for several days or even weeks. The parents frequently believe the discharge to represent an upper respiratory tract infection, thus explaining the delay. There may or may not be external excoriation around the nares.

The chief dangers of nasal foreign bodies are potential for aspiration, progression of local infection, and injury to the nose through clumsy removal of the foreign body.

In the case of the cooperative child, removal in the office may be tried. Good lighting and suction are essential. Cocaine, 10%, 2 to 3 drops, will frequently anesthetize the nose enough to allow insertion of a sucker or small nasal forceps. A #3 or #4 Fogarty catheter is also a useful and gentle tool if either the sucker or the forceps cannot grip the slippery object. For the uncooperative child, general anesthesia may be necessary. After removal of the foreign body, saline irrigations are frequently necessary for 2 or 3 days.

17 · *Drains*

WALTER J. PORIES, M.D.

Drains are often needed to evacuate fluid or pus from cavities or abscesses. Although they are often essential, especially if the space to be drained is deep and the opening narrow, they should be used sparingly and with caution. A drain is a foreign body in an infected space; it not only provides drainage but also allows other organisms to enter. Bacteria travel in both directions along drains. Drains are appropriately used only where a cavity with a small opening or a tract must be healed in from below.

PENROSE DRAINS

The drains most commonly used are the thin, floppy, flat rubber tubes known as Penrose drains. Supplied commercially in 1/4-, 1/2-, and 1-in widths and in 6- to 12-in lengths, they can be used singly or in pairs, in threes, or even in bunches.

1

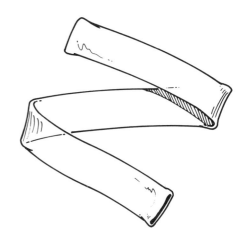

Penrose drains are overflow drains, in contrast to those that work by suction. Accordingly, they should, if possible, be placed to provide dependent drainage—that is, drainage out the most dependent portion of the wound. Penrose drains fall out of wounds easily and should therefore always be sutured in place. On occasion, they may also be sucked into the wound by respiratory or other muscular movements and have been reported as a cause of healing failure. To avoid this problem, surgeons not only suture a drain to a wound's edge but also transfix the protruding end with a safety pin.

2

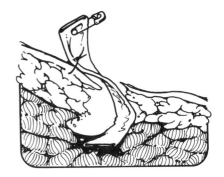

Penrose drains are usually left undisturbed for three to five days and then gradually advanced over another three to four days. Drains should not be disturbed until the drainage subsides substantially; when the dressings remain fairly dry, the drains can be advanced about 1 in each day. Drains should also be loosened or advanced if pain or fever arouses suspicion that drainage is not satisfactory.

If a Penrose drain is not immediately available, a serviceable substitute can be fabricated easily of a sterile rubber band or a suitable length cut from a sterile rubber glove. Penrose drains are also made of polyethylene and silicone, but there is no evidence that these more expensive models have any advantage over the plain rubber ones.

IODOFORM GAUZE

Iodoform gauze is occasionally used as a drain, but it is mentioned here only to condemn it.

3

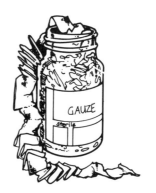

The material is unfortunately too easily available in most offices and emergency rooms and therefore continues to be used widely. It should *not* be used, however, for four reasons:

1. Iodoform is toxic to tissues and interferes with healing.

2. The gauze fills up the cavity and prevents the sides of the wound from collapsing (an important process essential for healing of abscesses).

3. The gauze dries out at the edge of the wound and forms a scab that seals the cavity.

4. The gauze causes pain on insertion, aggravates the pain because it prevents the escape of pus from the cavity, and hurts again when it is removed.

4

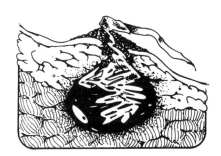

MALECOT CATHETERS

The Malecot catheter provides excellent drainage for small sinuses such as those associated with pilonidal sinuses, Bartholin's cysts, and fistulae in ano.

5

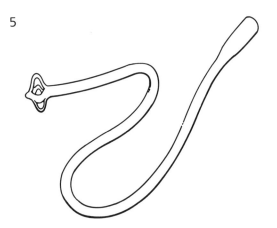

It can be inserted easily when it has been length-
ened and thinned with a clamp and will resume
its shape after withdrawal of the clamp. No
suture is needed because the catheter's bulbous
end keeps it in place. A safety pin through the
shaft of the catheter prevents its loss into the
cavity.

6a

6b

6c

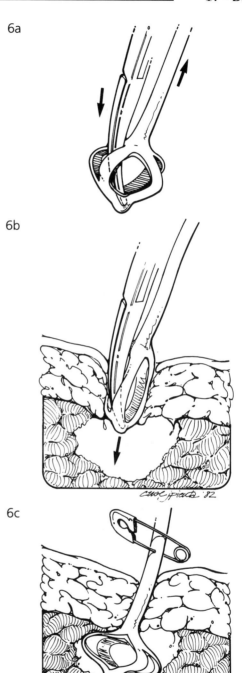

Malecot catheter drainage is well tolerated for long periods of time. In the military, we often drained pilonidal abscesses successfully with an incision only large enough to admit the catheter and were thus able to send patients back to duty the same day. The catheter can be removed when drainage becomes scant. It is withdrawn in the same manner as it was inserted: a clamp is inserted into the catheter and traction is applied to make it as thin as the opening.

FOLEY CATHETERS

If the abscess is too large for the Malecot catheter, or if the Malecot would be difficult to insert, as in some pararectal or ischiorectal abscesses, a Foley catheter can provide ideal drainage with little trauma. A suitably sized catheter (#14 to 20) with a 5- or 30-ml bag is gently inserted into the cavity through the drainage opening and inflated enough to keep it in place. The placement of the catheter can be checked with a roentgenogram, and most of the pus can be drained neatly into a plastic urine collection bag. The collapse of the abscess can be followed by serial sinograms if necessary; these are performed by injecting Hypaque or another water-soluble radio-opaque medium through the catheter. When the abscess has closed to the size of the Foley bag, the water in the balloon can be withdrawn gradually (about 10 ml every other day) and the catheter removed when the bag has collapsed.

7

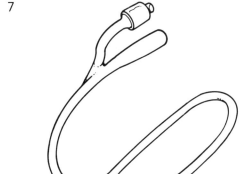

8

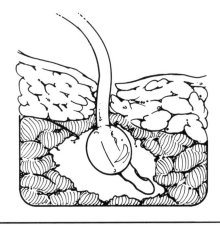

Foley balloons occasionally burst and allow the catheter to slip out of the sinus. To avoid this it is wise to fasten the catheter to the skin with a 3-0 suture.

SUMP CATHETERS

Sump catheters are rarely seen in office practice because they are usually used with continuous wall suction. Even so, they are included here for completeness and because patients are occasionally sent home with them. Sump catheters have two lumina, one of which is usually attached to suction, and the other serves as an air vent. A double-lumen catheter, such as a Salem sump, is also useful, however, for those cavities that may benefit from either constant or intermittent irrigation. Sumps can be used to clear wounds of clots or detritus and to instill antibiotics, chemotherapeutic agents, or other medications.

9

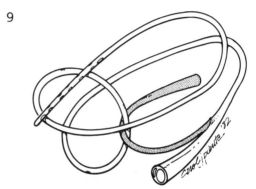

Because these plastic catheters are slippery and fall out easily, they need to be anchored with a suture of heavy 2-0 or 3-0 material. The suture is most effective if it is applied according to the principle of a Chinese finger trap—that is, not attached by a single tight tie about the tubing but wrapped loosely four or five times about the catheter. The technique is easier and far more secure.

SUCTION CATHETERS

Wound drainage catheters are occasionally attached to closed suction systems, which are
changed by compressing an elastic bulb and
which have the advantages of collapsing dead
space and draining the secretions neatly into a
container. This technique is especially useful for
drainage of wounds following operations such
as mastectomies, neck dissections, and thyro-
idectomies. We have been most pleased with
the Jackson-Pratt model because of its simplicity
and because it is made of Silastic and thus resists
clotting, but a large variety of products are available, and most of these seem to function well.
Although some miniaturized versions have been
developed for the office surgical market, these
do not seem, to us at least, to offer much prom-
ise.

10

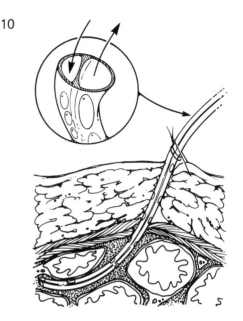

OBSTRUCTED DRAINAGE CATHETERS

Catheters become plugged all too readily, thus
changing their role from that of a conduit for
secretions to that of a foreign body in an undrained and infected cavity, producing sepsis
and pain. Occasionally a plugged catheter can
be opened with a flexible wire, but usually occlusion will recur shortly. Replacement of the
blocked catheter with a new one is better; if
the new tube is inserted immediately after withdrawal of the old, the same size can be used.
If the tube has been out even for several hours,
a smaller one will be indicated because of the
natural contraction of the tract.

REMOVAL OF THE DRAIN OR CATHETER

Drains should be removed as soon as they are no longer needed. For most cavities, this is the time when drainage has ceased or diminished sharply. In such cases, the drain should be loosened and advanced about 1 in; if little further exudate is seen, the drain can be removed.

In deep cavities, particularly those with tortuous, narrow, or long tracts, sinograms provide useful guidance. Sinograms are performed by injecting radio-opaque material such as Hypaque through the catheter so that the size, shape, location, and effectiveness of the drainage can be determined by roentgenography. The catheter is left in place as long as there is a sizable cavity; when this shrinks to a tube-shaped tract just larger than the drainage catheter, the catheter can be withdrawn slowly.

The drain site rarely requires more than a small dry dressing for a few days after the catheter or drain is removed; if it fails to heal, there is a good chance that an inadequately drained pocket still exists along the drainage tract.

18 · *Principles of Dressing Care*

WALTER J. PORIES, M.D.

Dressings are applied for many reasons. They can be designed to offer protection, to absorb blood secretions, to provide an environment for maceration and debridement, to apply medication, and to immobilize, support, and prevent edema. Dressings usually fulfill several of these functions simultaneously.

The dressing must be not only adapted to the wound but also appropriate for the patient's activities, economic situation, cultural beliefs, handicaps, and family situation, with consideration given to availability of materials. Because several kinds of dressings can ordinarily be used for any given situation, it is wise not to be rigid about their selection. For example, a dressing ideal for a farmer or soldier in the field would probably be inappropriate for a handicapped woman in her seventies.

Dressings require continuing evaluation. Be prepared to change a dressing quickly if it is painful or ineffective. Because large and complex dressings may be expensive and may interfere with daily activities, always strive to reduce their size, cost, and frequency of change whenever possible, and attempt to eliminate dressings altogether as soon as it is appropriate to do so.

Change dressings as infrequently as possible because dressing changes are painful, allow contamination, and are often a significant expense in hours and materials. In the past, wet dressings were changed every four hours or so to provide optimal wound cleansing, but the new wet occlusive dressing is much more effective and requires only one change daily. Similarly, dressings for absorption of purulent discharges may initially require changes every four hours to prevent overflow and seepage through the surface, but such drainage usually diminishes rapidly, and twice-a-day dressing changes can usually be initiated after 48 hr. Also, unless the patient has an unexplained fever or a tender wound surrounded by erythema or a rash, do not disturb a dry dressing applied in the operating room until the sutures are to be removed or until a dressing is no longer necessary. Some dressings are best left undisturbed for a long time: Unna paste can be left on for one to two weeks, and rigid plaster casts can remain intact

Table 1 Indications for Various Dressings

Wound	Dressing
Clean incisions, sutured lacerations	Dry dressing
Abrasions, rashes, superficial burns	Medicated dressing or Unna paste boot
Open debrided wounds	Dry occlusive dressing
Dirty, infected wounds with gangrene	Wet occlusive dressing
Infected space, abscess	Drain and absorbent dressing
Stasis ulcers, deep abrasions	Unna paste boot
Sprains and strains	Tape support, plaster casts
Bruises, sprains, contusions, rashes	Compresses

for several months. In some cases, prescribing frequent dressing changes can be helpful, as in helping a young mother work out her guilt for her child's injury through detailed and closely timed tasks that help reduce her anxiety.

Almost every commercial dressing can be replaced by an inexpensive alternative. Sanitary napkins cut into thirds make excellent absorbent dressings, and folded terry-cloth washcloths are effective reusable wet dressings. Elastic bandages can be used many times if properly cared for by frequent washings in cold water with a gentle cold-water soap like Woolite. The new Flexknit gauze tubing holds dressings as securely as gauze, with lower cost and less skin irritation.

Although a great variety of dressings are used throughout the world, the principles governing their use are universally accepted. Dressings are discussed here in relation to their indications; they are also summarized in Table 1.

DRY DRESSINGS

The ideal dressing for clean incisions and lacerations protects them from contact with extraneous bacteria, cushions touch, absorbs the small amount of tissue ooze, and provides an aesthetic cover.

1

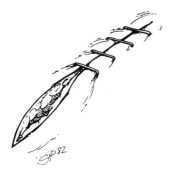

2

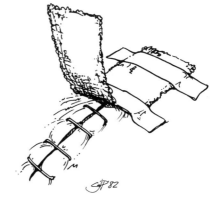

After 48 hr a dry dressing usually can be removed and the wound left exposed, or, better, the wound can be covered with a single layer of one of the new tapes made of plastic or paper. The single layer of tape is cosmetically acceptable and inexpensive, protects the sutures or staples from catching, and provides considerable comfort for the patient. We highly recommend Micropore paper tape or similar products, which adhere well when wet, allowing the patient to bathe and to wash directly over the healing wound. We frequently replace the tape after the sutures are removed, leaving it in place for two or three more weeks; this approach provides better continued support of the wound edges during healing and seems to produce finer scars. Patients can purchase Micropore tape readily and replace it themselves if it loosens or becomes soiled.

3

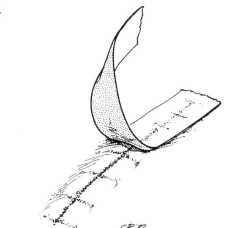

4

MEDICATED DRESSINGS FOR ABRASIONS, RASHES, AND SUPERFICIAL BURNS

5

Abrasions, rashes, and superficial burns hurt or itch when exposed to air, frequently ooze, become infected easily, are unsightly, and are liable to be picked or scratched by the ailing patient. Therefore, the dressing should exclude air, bacteria, and probing fingers and should be absorbent and neat in appearance.

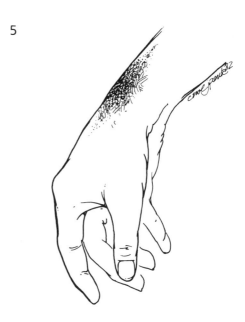

6

A dressing with three layers is extremely effective. The bottom layer consists of one sheet of fine-mesh gauze impregnated with any of a variety of ointments or salves to minimize infection and sticking. We prefer Betadine ointment at this time but have used Furacin, Neosporin, Bacitracin, and Vaseline gauze with good results. For burns, mafenide (Sulfamylon) cream is widely used.

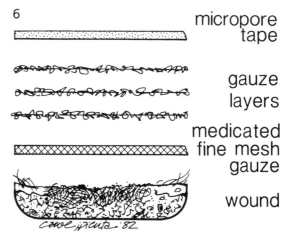

micropore tape

gauze layers

medicated fine mesh gauze

wound

Absorption is provided by two or three additional layers of 4- × 4-in gauze, and the dressing is finally sealed and held in place with tape.

7

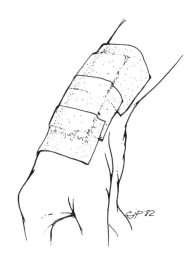

As in most types of dressings, variations are possible. In the absence of medicated fine-mesh gauze, apply the ointment directly to the wound and cover it with dry fine-mesh gauze (inexpensive and widely available as roll gauze).

8

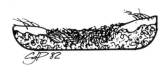

roll gauze

fine mesh gauze

ointment

wound

For the extremities, we prefer Kerlix or Kling to tape for holding the dressing in place.

9

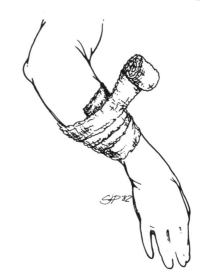

To fasten dressings for large lesions of the trunk, we strongly recommend Flexknit, an inexpensive elastic mesh supplied in tubes of various sizes; this product does not irritate (as does tape), facilitates dressing changes, and accommodates comfortably to the patient's body.

10

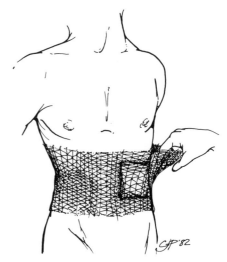

OCCLUSIVE DRY DRESSINGS FOR OPEN,
CONTAMINATED WOUNDS

The treatment of contaminated wounds from
injuries such as explosions, tissue avulsions, industrial crushing accidents, and shotgun wounds
has been markedly improved through the experience and studies of the military. Debride
such wounds diligently until all dead tissue, detritus, clots, and contaminants have been removed (see Chapter 9).

11

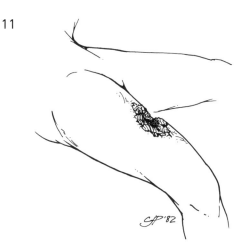

At the end of the debridement, no crushed or
questionably viable tissue should remain, tissues
must bleed readily when cut, muscles should
contract, and blood vessels, tendons, bones,
joints, and nerves should all be covered by viable
tissue.

12

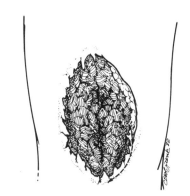

When debridement is complete, first cover the wound with a *single* layer of moistened fine-mesh gauze carefully placed to fill each of the hollows and crevices.

13

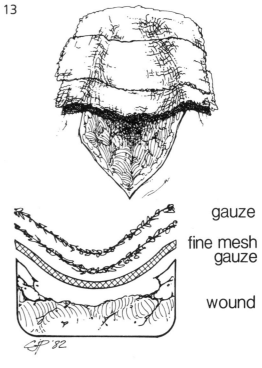

gauze

fine mesh gauze

wound

Fill the wound with a large amount of absorptive fluffed gauze or vaginal packs so that the cavity is voluminously filled.

14

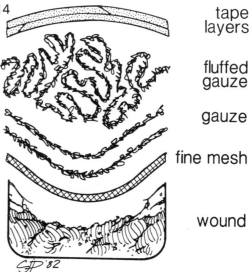

tape layers

fluffed gauze

gauze

fine mesh

wound

Although such debridement is usually best done in an operating room under general anesthesia, small wounds can often be handled in an emergency room or office. Similarly, a disaster or an accident in a remote site may require debridement under less than ideal conditions. Whatever the situation, however, adhere to the principles of thorough debridement because the final cleanliness of the wound is far more important than the condition of the facility.

Make the dressing occlusive by covering it with a complete layer of tape. Painting the skin immediately surrounding the wound with tincture of benzoin before applying the tape helps to protect the skin and to promote adhesion.

15

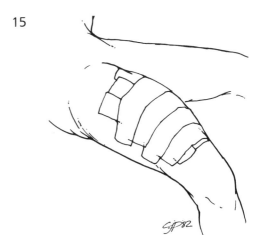

Leave the dressing undisturbed for four to five days to maintain sterility and to allow early granulation. Invade the dressing only if there is excessive bleeding or if signs of local or systemic infection appear.

On the fourth or fifth day following the injury, remove the dressing under sterile precautions (with masks and gloves), and carefully examine the wound. If the entire wound is odorless, clean, free of necrosis, and showing early granulation, close it with sutures, cover it with a graft, or treat it by a combination of these two approaches. We emphasize the so-called golden period of four to six days for the dressing change and secondary closure. Infection and breakdown are more likely to occur if the wound is closed earlier than this; if it is closed later, the edges may be retracted and rigid, making closure difficult and the wound more susceptible to infection.

We normally use 2-0 Prolene on large cutting-edge needles for approximation of the wound edges and can usually close most wounds.

The grafts, if needed, are thin split-thickness (10/1,000 to 13/1,000 in) for maximum take and contracture. Such grafts can be cut with a disposable, plastic, battery-powered derma-tome, a hand dermatome, or even a sterile razor blade held by a straight clamp. Fix the grafts in place with 4-0 braided suture, staples, or paper tape.

16

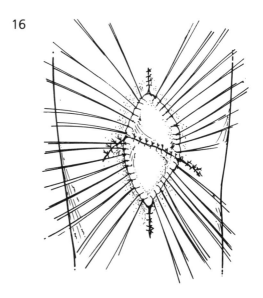

A stent (a ball of cotton shaped to provide even compression throughout the wound) holds the grafts in place. Prepare the stent by covering the grafts with a single layer of fine-mesh gauze medicated with Furacin or Betadine and filling the cavity with layers of moist cotton until the cotton heaps about 1 to 2 cm above the surface of the graft. Tie the ends of the sutures securing the graft over the cotton in opposing pairs to hold the dressing securely.

17

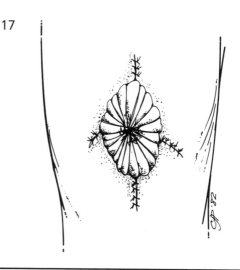

18

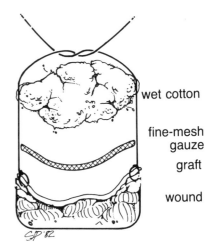

wet cotton

fine-mesh
gauze

graft

wound

The final dressing consists of dry gauze and
Kerlix, Kling, or Flexknit to protect the suture
lines and the stent. Examine the stent daily after
the third day following its application. If the
dressing emits no foul odor, the grafts are probably healing well and should be left undisturbed
for seven to ten days. If there is an odor about
the wound (and this is not a subtle change—
it will be foul), the grafts are infected and the
stent should be promptly removed.

19

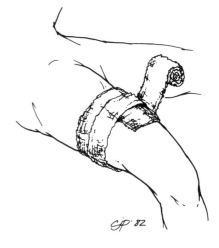

Remove the stent by soaking it with saline
washes from an Asepto syringe for 10 to 15
min, cutting the sutures, and removing it delicately with constant irrigation to avoid lifting
the grafts from the wound. Patience here is
amply rewarded.

20

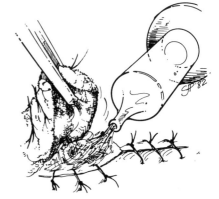

Grafts need to be supported by external pressure during the first month or two because their vasculature is delicate and a sudden shock or blow may cause bleeding under the graft and its subsequent loss. A good approach is to cover the graft with several layers of soft rubber or plastic sponge, holding the cushion in place with an elastic bandage or an elastic stocking.

21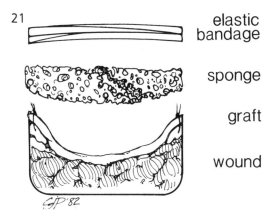

elastic
bandage

sponge

graft

wound

WET OCCLUSIVE, OR EARLE, DRESSINGS FOR DIRTY, INFECTED WOUNDS WITH GANGRENOUS TISSUE

Infected wounds are common, especially among diabetic patients with neuropathic feet. Such wounds are also seen in inadequately cared-for gunshot injuries, in decubitus ulcers, infected crush injuries, and other similar conditions.

22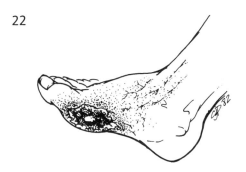

Patients with such wounds are often septic and critically ill. In addition to local treatment of the wound, such patients need bed rest, fluids, and two or three antibiotic drugs given intravenously. We use penicillin and chloramphenicol, gentamicin and cefamandole, cefoxitin and cefazolin, or clindamycin, tobramycin, and cefazolin.

It is essential to rule out ischemia from atherosclerosis or other vascular diseases because, in cases of inadequate blood supply, healing will not occur without vascular reconstruction (if reconstruction is not possible, amputation is usually necessary). Similarly, a deep abscess or undrained pocket should always be suspected and sought with needle aspiration and a sinogram. If an abscess is found, it must be drained adequately but conservatively; enthusiastic manipulation may break down natural barriers, encourage spread of infection, and extend the gangrene.

An excellent approach to these difficult wounds is the wet occlusive dressing designed to macerate and debride the gangrenous tissues. It is sometimes known as the Earle dressing, after the plastic surgeon who first described it.

First cover the wound with a moistened layer of fine-mesh gauze placed so it fills and lies in contact with each crevice and hollow of the wound. Then carefully lay a thick layer of wet fluffed 4 × 4s over the fine-mesh gauze to ensure good contact of the gauze with every portion of the wound and to provide adequate absorption.

Snugly apply a wrap of Kerlix or Kling to ensure good contact between the tissues and the gauze and to avoid an air interface that will interfere with the maceration. Two rolls are usually needed.

23

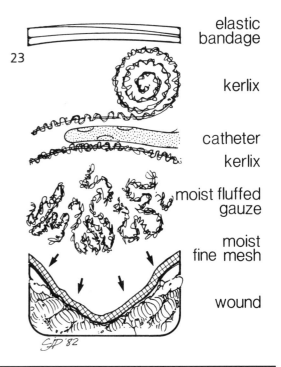

elastic
bandage

kerlix

catheter
kerlix

moist fluffed
gauze

moist
fine mesh

wound

24

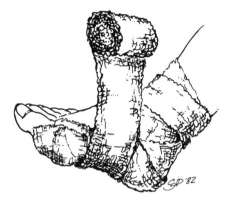

Keep the dressing moist with a catheter attached to a bottle of normal saline solution. Incorporate the #14 French catheter into the dressing by including it into the wraps of Kling or Kerlix.

The last layer of the dressing consists of two rolls of elastic bandage wrapped snugly to ensure good tissue contact. This thick elastic bandage also helps maintain moisture within the dressing.

25

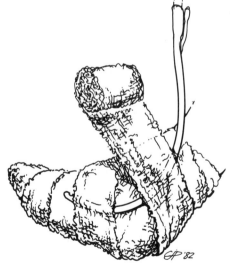

26

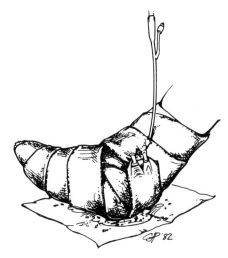

Initiate the saline drip at a rapid rate until the fluid runs out the bottom of the bandage. Then slow the drip and keep the dressing moist to the touch around the clock by adjustment of the drip. The adjustment of the drip does not have to be done by a nurse; patients and families can easily be taught to do this, even at home.

The dressing should be changed only once a day, preferably by the physician, to debride the softened, macerated tissues. If the wound is kept wet, the necrotic tissues will liquefy. If the wound becomes dry, the dressing either has not been kept wet enough or was not applied snugly, leaving an air interface between the dressing and the tissue surfaces. Limit debridement *only* to the clearly dead, grey, mushy tissue. If correctly done, the procedure should be painless, and there should be no bleeding. Patience and gentleness are rewarded. Too-aggressive debridement encourages excessive tissue loss, progressive necrosis, and sepsis and is cruel to the patient.

27

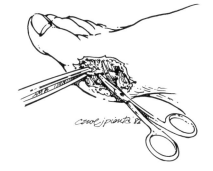

Most wounds can be cleansed totally within five days, but in unusually deep wounds or in the case of diabetic patients, this cleansing may take a few more days.

When the wound is pink and granulating well, it can be grafted or allowed to heal in slowly. At this stage a dry medicated dressing (discussed earlier) or an Unna paste boot (discussed later) usually suffices.

DRESSING A WOUND WITH A DRAIN

Dressing care of a wound with a drain—for example, after the drainage of an abscess—is directed toward absorption of the purulent material from the wound and maintenance of drainage by keeping the environment moist to prevent scab formation. The dressings are frequently made occlusive to diminish the chances of spreading the organism and to protect clothing.

28

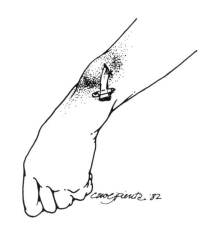

For absorption, cover the abscess with a layer of 4 × 4s and one or several abdominal pads, which are then held in place by a Kerlix or Kling covering.

29

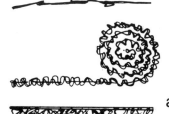

plastic

Kling
or Kerlix

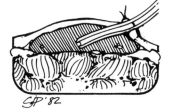

abdominal
pads

gauze

drain

abscess

The dressings can be covered with a layer of plastic from a wastebasket liner or a dry cleaner's bag to maintain the moist environment and to protect clothing and furniture.

30

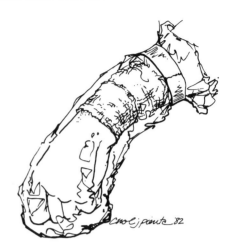

Initially, the dressings can be dry because the purulent secretions provide moisture. During this time, change the dressing frequently enough to maintain a clean outer layer; dressing changes every 4 to 6 hr will usually suffice. After 2 to 3 days the dressing may need to be moistened to prevent scabbing. After 4 to 5 days, the drain can be removed and a small dry dressing applied.

UNNA PASTE BOOT FOR STASIS ULCERS

Stasis ulcers are common afflictions that often receive poor treatment. Patients frequently arrive in the surgeon's office in tears, exhausted from lack of sleep and continuing pain. They are usually incredulous when told that the ulcer, which frequently extends down to bone, can be healed without surgery and that only special dressing care is needed.

31

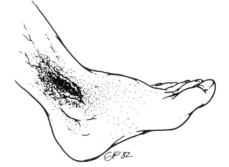

Dressing care with an Unna paste boot (Dohme's paste) for stasis ulcers provides for the direct application of the impregnated calamine cream (an ancient medication containing zinc oxide) to the wound and the control of edema with the inelastic support bandage.

32

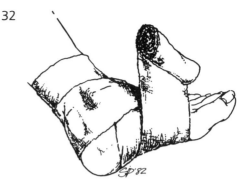

Before applying the bandage, gently wash the foot and the ulcer with soap and water or Betadine solution, avoiding any discomfort to the patient. Do not debride or scrub the ulcer, and *do not apply a dressing* under the bandage. Rather, apply the Unna paste bandage directly to the ulcer and the skin. Wrapping the Unna paste boot requires practice; the inelastic bandage needs a tuck at almost every turn to make it conform to the leg. It requires firm and snug application to control the edema yet should not interfere with circulation.

A single layer of Kerlix is wrapped over the freshly applied boot to protect the patient's clothing from soiling by the drying paste. The boot will usually be dry within 24 hr, and the Kerlix covering can then be removed.

33

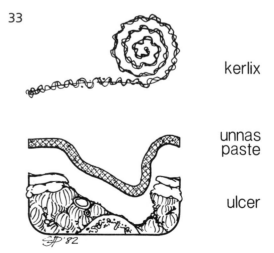

kerlix

unnas paste

ulcer

The bandage is best applied in the morning before the leg has had a chance to swell. A dose of 40 mg of Lasix the night before also helps minimize edema.

Patients can walk immediately in the boot, but frequently it will not fit into their shoe. Advise them to bring in slippers, sandals, or an old shoe that can be cut if necessary.

Some families can be taught to change the Unna paste bandages; when healing is well underway they welcome the chance to make such a contribution, and this should be encouraged.

Because the Unna paste boot is a wonderfully absorptive bandage, warn the patient that secretions from the ulcer are expected to soak into the bandage and that areas of discoloration that may even stay moist will appear. Emphasize that these are good signs that indicate the dressing is doing its job.

Even with excellent dressing care, stasis ulcers heal slowly. It is not unusual for them to require two to four months for complete repair. When the ulcer has healed, switch the patient to strong elastic hose and advise him or her that such elastic support may be needed for many years to come. Recurrent and intractable stasis ulcers are usually due to a large so-called feeding vein (a misnomer because it is really an incompetent vein that interferes with venous drainage).

TAPING JOINTS AFTER SPRAINS

Sprains are ligamentous tears, usually produced by overextension of the joint. Mild sprains can be helped by taping, but the procedure is very much inferior to casting. We mention it here for completeness and advise it only in situations where a cast may be unacceptable, such as on a hike or bivouac when casting materials may not be available or when the injury is relatively minor.

34

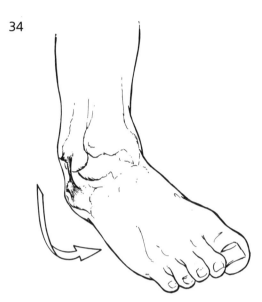

After the examination has pinpointed the damaged ligament, flex the joint in the direction of the sprain to take the pull off the ligament.

35

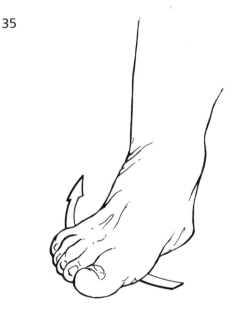

Apply 1-in tape tightly in a basketweave pattern, parallel to the direction of the damaged fibers. Several applications of tincture of benzoin will protect the skin and aid adhesion, and an elastic bandage over the tape may help to reduce edema.

36

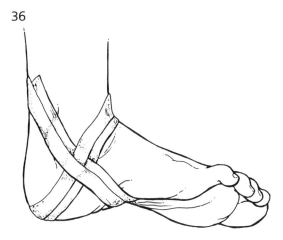

PLASTER CASTS

Fractures, sprains, strains, and various other problems are best treated with a cast. There are many ways to apply a cast and many casting materials, including thermosetting plastics, but for the practitioner who does not apply a large number of casts, the stockinette-Webril/rapid-cast plaster technique described here is safe, effective, dependable, and inexpensive. A below-knee cast is described as an example.

The ideal cast is light, of even thickness throughout, not too tight or too loose, and without indentations, which can cause pressure sores. With considerable practice it is possible to form an excellent below-knee cast using no more than two rolls of plaster.

While wrapping the cast, take care to keep the extremity in a position of function. For most ankle injuries the ankle should be at 90 degrees of flexion without eversion or inversion.

37

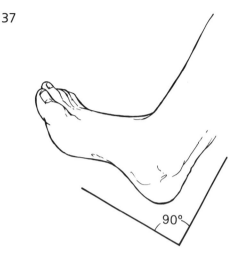

The patient can help maintain this position by holding up the ends of a strip of bandage looped under the toe, just as he or she would hold a horse's rein.

38

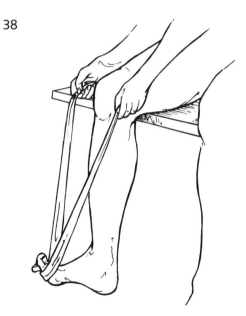

First, slip a stockinette of suitable size onto the leg, pull it up to the knee, and smooth it free of wrinkles. Then wrap Webril (a bandage made of compressed cotton) around the leg in two or three layers, tearing it as needed to make it conform smoothly to the leg. The Webril should extend almost to the knee and to the toes including the heel.

39

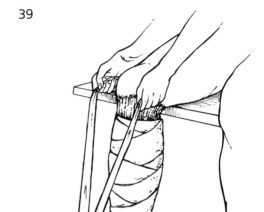

Next, apply the plaster. We prefer the rapid-setting material. Immerse a 4-in roll in warm water until no further bubbles escape from the plaster. Gently squeeze excess water from the roll and begin the wrap. It is easier to work with a slightly dripping wet bandage than a heavily squeezed one.

40

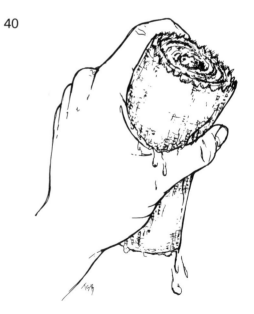

The toes are much less likely to be injured if a tongue of plaster is prepared with four to six thicknesses of plaster strips to protrude for a half inch or so beyond their tips. The extension also provides support to the toes and gives them a surface to press against for exercise.

41

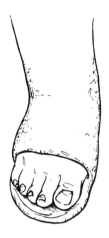

Casts should be supported while drying. If allowed merely to rest on a flat surface, they will flatten and dry in an unsatisfactory shape. Therefore, provide the needed support with the flat of the hands for about 10 min, avoiding using the fingertips and moving the hands frequently to prevent indentations.

To give a cast a professional appearance, polish and harden the final layer of the plaster by smoothing it constantly as it dries. If desired, a high polish can easily be achieved by buffing the almost-dry cast with green soap.

To finish the top and bottom of the cast, fold the excess stockinette over the cast, cover it with a wet strip of plaster, and smooth it into place.

42

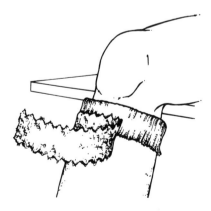

Practicing on an irregular object such as a crooked tree limb helps the physician develop smoothness in laying the plaster, which is best achieved by unrolling it with the left hand while forming tucks and smoothing with the right hand. When the cast is dry, cut it from the practice object and examine it for uniformity of thickness and strength. (It is best to practice in a fenced-in backyard so you don't undermine your neighbors' confidence in your skills!)

43

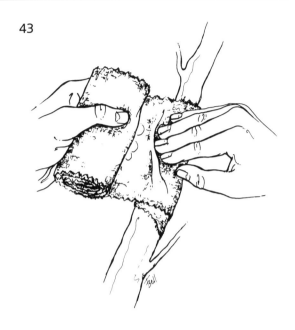

The full-length leg casts are best constructed as composites; the below-knee portion is formed as described (except that the stockinette and Webril extend to the groin) and is allowed to harden before wrapping the knee. This approach makes the job of controlling joints much easier and ensures a better final cast.

44

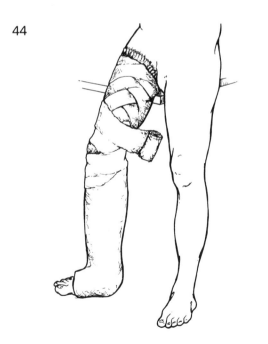

In casting the hand and forearm, unless there are specific contraindications such as a Colles' or other complex fracture, pay attention to dorsiflexing the wrist and allowing for maximum mobility of the fingers in the position of function (that used in grasping a baseball—that is, with the wrist in extension and the metacarpophalangeal joints at 90 degrees of flexion). This position can be achieved easily by letting the cast extend no further than the proximal crease of the hand and by allowing an opening for the thumb large enough to permit opposition to the little finger.

45

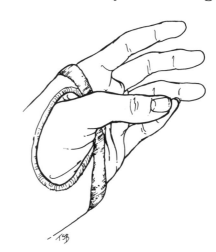

Casts can produce severe ischemic injury. Complications from ill-fitting, tight casts are a frequent cause of litigation. Even if a cast is quite loose at the time of application, increasing edema or the development of a hematoma can produce dangerous encroachment. Accordingly, observe patients closely after the application of casts, and check them for swelling, pain, anesthesia, fever, decreased vascular supply to the digits, and inability to move the intrinsic muscles of the hand or foot over the following 8 to 12 hr. Instruct the patient and his or her family both orally and in writing how to check for problems and to notify the physician if they have concerns.

If there is evidence of ischemia or suspicion of localized pressure that might produce local necrosis, regard the situation as a medical emergency and treat the patient without delay. Even an hour or two is sufficient for development of causalgia, Volkmann's contracture, or gangrene. In such cases, either split (bivalve) the cast or remove it. In splitting or bivalving a cast, divide the cast *all the way down to skin.* Blood-coated Webril or taut stockinette forms just as effective a tourniquet as plaster. Unless skin is exposed for the entire length of the cast, it is difficult to be certain that the problem has been solved. Putting on a new cast is always preferable to worrying about a questionable one.

46

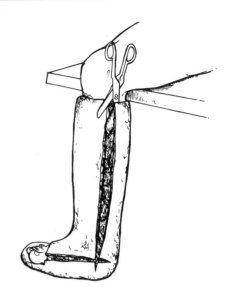

Patients are normally comfortable if they keep a casted extremity elevated on one or two pillows for the first 24 hr. This measure decreases edema and diminishes venous ooze and hematoma formation.

If weight bearing is to be permitted, attach a rubber walking heel to the cast the next day. Reinforce the sole of the cast with six to eight layers of plaster splints, and attach the rubber heel with additional plaster bandages.

47

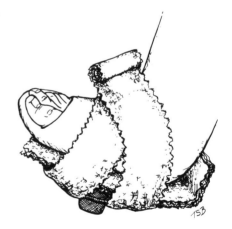

Patients may have difficulty maneuvering with a cast, especially if they are frail or have had no previous experience with crutches. Such patients may benefit greatly from training with a physical therapist for one or more sessions.

Ordinary plaster casts will soften with moisture and therefore need protection during bathing or exposure to rain or snow. For the easiest approach, insert the casted limb into one or two plastic dry cleaners' bags or garbage bags, closing off the tops with two or three rubber bands. This arrangement is not completely waterproof but does allow the patient to take a quick shower or to get about in bad weather.

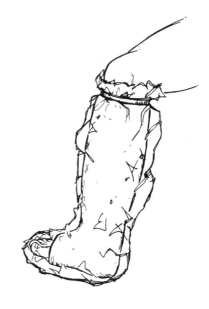

A sling can provide considerable comfort to a patient with a casted upper extremity. It relieves the arm of the weight of the cast, minimizes edema, and encourages use of the hand. Slings can be made of strips of bandage, but they are best fashioned from a large triangle of muslin tied behind the neck and pinned to provide a pocket for the elbow. Ready-made slings of sturdy cloth and adjustable woven tapes can also be used. All should be washable.

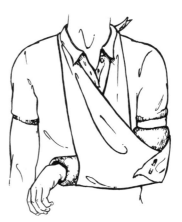

COMPRESSES

Hot and cold compresses are useful adjuncts for a number of minor problems such as bruises, sprains, and skin eruptions. They greatly enhance comfort and carry little, if any, risk (if excesses in temperature are avoided).

The guidelines for hot versus cold compresses remain unclear. Arguments have raged for centuries, but most practitioners agree that cold compresses prevent swelling and absorption of toxins, while hot compresses help to resolve cellulitis, hasten absorption of superficial clots, help bring abscesses to a head, and soothe the pains of neuritis, myositis, and arthritis.

Compresses can be applied over a cutaneous counterirritant such as Vick's Vaporub or Absorbine Jr. but usually consist of a simple absorptive bandage moistened with water or a solution of Epsom salts. Wet, thick, terry-cloth toweling (washcloths will do) may be used, covered by either an electric heating pad, a hot-water bottle, or a bag of ice. A plastic bag or wrap placed about and under the compress helps maintain the temperature and protects furniture and clothing. The temperature should be monitored closely; it is easy to produce significant burns, especially in children and in patients under medication. Never use such treatment on a sleeping or unconscious patient.

SALVES, SOLUTIONS, OINTMENTS, AND
OTHER TOPICAL MEDICATIONS

A wide variety of topical medications is available for office treatment of surgical problems. We question whether there are great differences among these products and have chosen, therefore, to list in Table 2 only those we use frequently and have found helpful.

50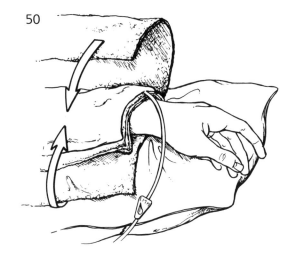

Table 2 Topical Medications

Purpose	Agent
Cleansing and preparation of skin	Betadine soap or paint, hexachlorophene
Removal of scabs and dried clots from a wound or graft	3% hydrogen peroxide
Irrigation of a wound or sinus to clear it of clots or pus	Water or saline (with addition of approximately 0.5 gm kanamycin per 1,000 ml of solution)
Prevention of infection and lubrication in presence of indwelling catheter (such as a catheter in the common duct, the subclavian vein, etc.)	Betadine ointment under occlusive dressing
Prevention of infection and sticking in granulating wound	Betadine ointment, Furacin gauze, Neosporin-Bacitracin ointment, Op-Site
Promotion of granulation	Scarlet-red-impregnated gauze
Control of infection and odor in an indolent wound, decubitus ulcer, cavity, or ulcerating tumor	Balsam of Peru, half-strength Dakin's solution, Debrisan granules
Protection of skin under tape	Tincture of benzoin
Protection of skin from effects of a fistula or ostomy	Aluminum paste, A & D ointment, Karaya gum powder
Scaling and drying of skin, especially in areas previously irradiated, in frail or undernourished patients, and near wet dressings	Crisco (far better than cocoa butter and other expensive creams and better than other brands)

Note: For rashes and other dermatologic disorders, the reader is referred to the dermatologic literature.

19 · *Bandaging Techniques*

WALTER J. PORIES, M.D.

Patients expect to leave their doctor's office with a neat, comfortable bandage, but such bandages may, on occasion, be difficult to apply. One of the oldest aphorisms still works: If the dressing doesn't look nice, just add more bandage. It is often surprising to see an apparently hopeless dressing become a beautiful bandage with application of only a few more turns of Kerlix or Kling.

Innovation and common sense are important in dressing care. Stockinette makes an excellent head dressing when knotted into a cap, a bra lined with gauze becomes an ideal breast dressing, and a corset or abdominal binder can hold an absorbent dressing better than multiple applications of tape. Each of these is an adaptation of readily available materials. Several common bandaging techniques for various parts of the body are illustrated in this chapter.

HEAD

Although many books illustrate the technique of dressing the head with a roll bandage, this method is used infrequently today because such dressings rarely stay in place. Moreover, if wrapped or taped too tightly to the skull, they can produce a circular area of necrosis at the level of a hatband.

Four other widely used approaches to bandaging the head are illustrated. The most useful and aesthetically acceptable for adults is the disposable surgical cap. It is not unattractive and is disposable, inexpensive, readily available and, if the rim is folded upward and tied, capable of holding a dressing securely in place.

1

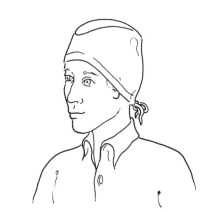

For small children, the knotted tube stockinette or tube Flexknit with a hole cut for the face works well, is well tolerated, and does not become dislodged during play. The edges fray surprisingly little, and taping of the opening is not needed.

2

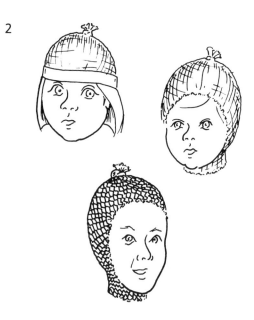

FINGERS

Bandages with roll gauze are rarely used today because they are often bulky and easily dislodged during manual tasks. Even so, the roll gauze method is illustrated for completeness and because there are occasions when only a gauze roll is available.

Finger Dressing with Gauze Roll

3

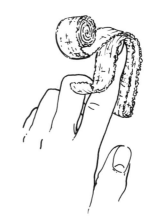

Fold the 1-in gauze over the tip of the finger several times to cover and cushion the lesion.

Wrap the gauze around the folds in spirals up and down the finger several times until the bandage is neat and feels secure. A sloppy, loose bandage usually means not enough gauze was used, and additional turns should be taken.

4

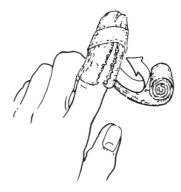

Secure the bandage by tying it about the wrist. To do so, first draw the gauze down along the back of the hand to beyond the wrist. With this technique the gauze does not get caught in the palm. Then split the end beyond the wrist lengthwise with scissors up to the level of the wrist.

5

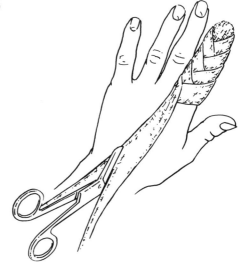

Tie the two tails in a knot at the level of the wrist and bring them around the wrist and tie again.

6

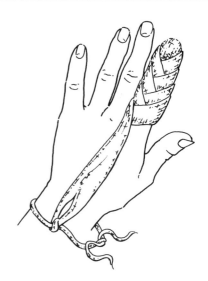

If two or three fingers require bandaging, they all can be incorporated into a dressing of this kind, but several layers of gauze should be interposed between the fingers as a cushion and to absorb perspiration and tissue fluids.

Finger Dressing with Tube Gauze

The tube gauze method of dressing fingers is rapid, gentle to the patient, and inexpensive. It provides an excellent, secure, absorbent, and aesthetically satisfying dressing. We regard it as the method of choice.

Draw the tube gauze of the appropriate size over the metal cage provided with the product (if the metal cage has been lost, an aluminum splint bent into a U will do as well or even a large test tube or centrifuge tube can serve).

7

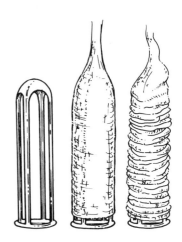

Gently insert the finger into the cage and draw the gauze onto the finger. Guide the gauze past the slippery metal onto the skin. 8

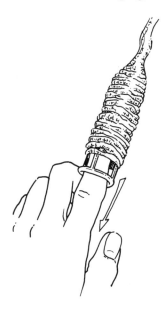

Gently withdraw the cage through the open end of the tube gauze, leaving the first layer of the gauze on the finger. Twist the gauze 360 degrees to form a spiral seal at the tip, invert the end, and pull it over the finger again to form the second layer. 9

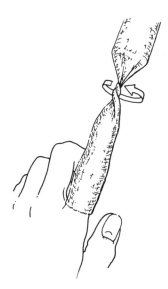

Place three to four layers of gauze on the finger. When enough tube gauze has been deposited on the finger, slit the excess longitudinally on both sides of the finger to the base to form two strips of gauze. Then knot these two strips and tie them around the wrist to secure the dressing.

10

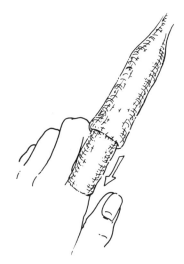

11

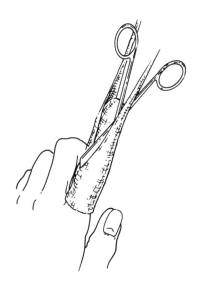

12

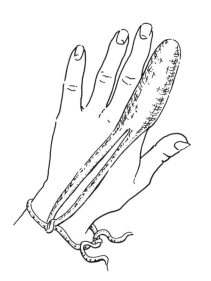

Finger Dressing with Elastoplast or Other
Adherent Bandage

Finger dressings with elastic adhesive bandages
are easy to apply and are neat in appearance
but are less secure than tube gauze. However,
for short-term dressings they serve well.

Cover the lesion with a small sponge. Wrap a
piece of Elastoplast or similar product around
the finger and trim the excess about 5 mm away
from the finger.

13

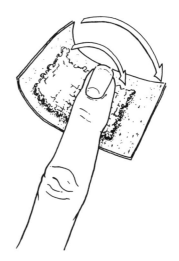

14

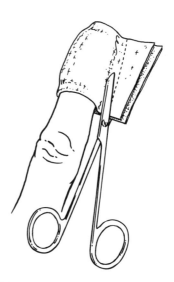

The final bandage is surprisingly waterproof. The dressing works well for patients with manual jobs. Such patients, if given a roll of Elastoplast, can easily replace the bandage, should it become loose or unsightly.

15

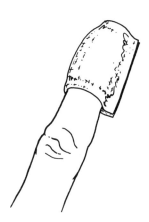

ARMS AND LEGS

Dressings for the limbs are not difficult to apply, but they must be snug enough to stay on yet not so tight that they act as a tourniquet. If the skin is painted with several layers of tincture of benzoin before the dressing is applied, the gauze will adhere much better to the sticky skin.

Rather than regular gauze, use elastic gauze such as Kerlix or Kling, which accommodates nicely to limbs and stretches easily, making a tourniquet effect less likely.

Initially, anchor the bandage by closely overlapping the first layers. Wrap the bandage in a figure-of-8 spiral to produce overlapping, interweaving, and self-locking layers, for a neat and secure final bandage.

16

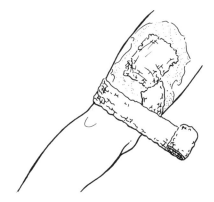

17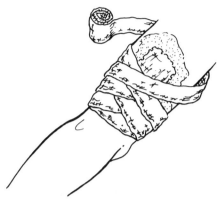

Usually a piece of tape suffices to secure the end of the gauze roll.

18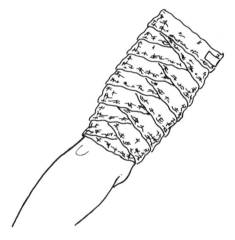

In active patients, several spirals of 1-in tape add strength to the dressing. Apply the tape only as a spiral, never as a circle, because the tape can act as a tourniquet. Use no tape on the skin; it is not needed and may cause considerable irritation.

19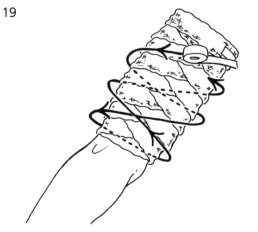

Extremities

20

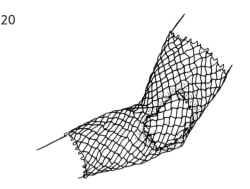

An easy, inexpensive, and effective dressing for the extremities can be made with Flexknit or similar tubular dressing material. These materials come in various sizes, ranging from a small size, appropriate for a finger dressing, to tubes large enough to dress the thorax. Simply cut the material to size and carefully slip it over the dressing. No tape is needed. The material can be used for a surprisingly long time, and the dressing underneath can be changed many times a day without changing the Flexknit wrapper.

Hands

21

Dress the hand in a position of function, as if it were about to catch an orange:

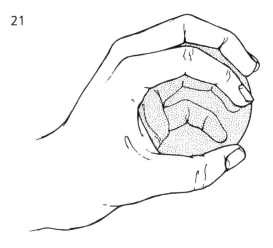

- The wrist is extended.

- The MP joints are at 90 to 100 degrees of flexion.

- The fingers are separated by about 0.5 cm.

- The thumb is in opposition to and about 10 cm from the little finger.

The importance of the position of function cannot be overemphasized. Hands become stiff very easily. If the hand is not bandaged properly, a flexed wrist, straightened MP joints, and subluxed finger joints may be the early result. Such hands are almost impossible to rehabilitate. Even with minimal movement, a hand in the position of function can carry out many tasks. The neglected hand can do little and in fact may never again be able to do much. Such tragedies are preventable. Closely monitor patients with hand injuries, and institute a physiotherapy program early.

Place gauze between all the fingers to separate and cushion them. A cock-up splint for the wrist helps maintain it in dorsiflexion. The splint can be fabricated easily with about four to six layers of wet 3-in plaster bandage, cushioned by a layer or two of gauze bandage, or a commercial aluminum splint may be used.

22

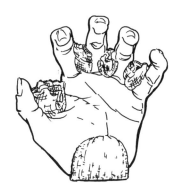

Build up a bulky wrap of Kerlix about the hand and between the fingers to about the first PIP joint, until only the fingertips protrude. This dressing allows minimal activity and provides a means for evaluating the tightness of the dressing; the fingers can be checked easily for intact sensation, color, motion, and capillary return.

23

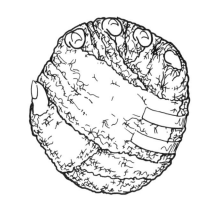

Most patients with hand dressings benefit from a sling because the dressing is often heavy and bulky.

24

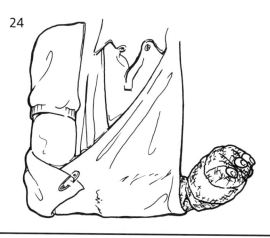

Hand dressings can usually be left undisturbed for 5 to 10 days unless they become malodorous or unsightly or unless pain or signs of generalized sepsis appear.

Hands stiffen easily (it's worth repeating), so function and motion should be resumed as early as possible.

Feet and Legs

Dry Bandages   Dressings can be held in place on the lower extremity with Kerlix, Kling, and elastic bandages. Kerlix and Kling are absorbent soft gauze bandages that accommodate easily to the contours of the foot and leg. Elastic bandages can be either nonadherent (Ace) or adherent (Elastoplast). Occasionally the two types are used in combination, with the Kerlix or Kling to cushion and absorb and the elastic, thick, rubberized wraps to minimize edema and protect the wound from dirt.

Apply one or several coats of tincture of benzoin on the skin to keep the bandage from slipping.

To anchor the bandage, take one turn about the foot at the insole, bring the bandage up around the ankle, and then return to wrap the foot, beginning just behind the toes. The bandage should be layered in a figure-of-8 fashion to optimize contact between the layers for anchoring and neatness. Finally, make one or two flat turns at the top of the bandage for a finished appearance.

When two bandages are required because of inadequate length of each roll, anchor the first to itself with tape or clips. Then begin the second roll at the same place, anchoring it with an extra flat wrap or two, and continue the progress of the wrap as shown.

27

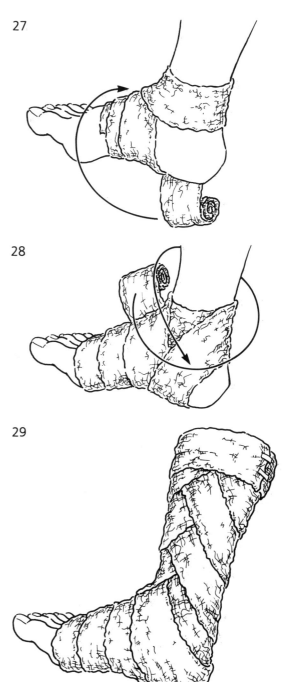

25

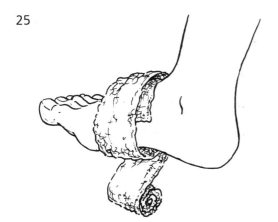

28

26

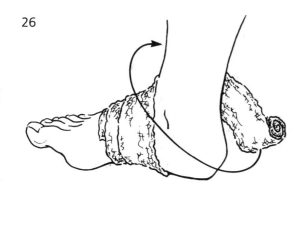

29

Unna Boot   The Unna boot is described in detail on pp. 230–232. In essence, it is an ancient dressing dating back to the time of the Egyptians, consisting of a thin, inelastic muslin wrap coated with calamine (zinc oxide) ointment. The bandage is applied like a cast but directly over skin and open sores, if any are present. Because it is inelastic, it controls edema; the zinc is thought to promote healing. An Unna boot dries to a soft, pliable cast that is well tolerated and that allows patients to carry on their usual daily activities and return to their jobs. It is normally changed once a week and is easily removed with bandage scissors.

We use the Unna boot often, especially for conditions such as chronic lesions of the legs, mild sprains, venous ulcers, superficial burns, and neurodermatitis.

CHEST AND TRUNK

The gauze wrap method of dressing the trunk is no longer used widely because of the superiority and wide availability of Flexknit. We include it here, however, for completeness.

Begin the gauze wrap with the help of the patient or an assistant to steady the dressing and the end of the bandage. We prefer Kerlix or Kling to plain gauze because of its elasticity.

30

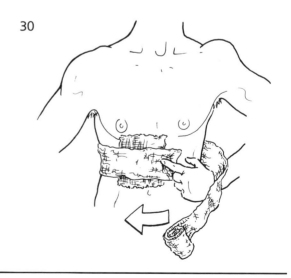

Take several turns around the trunk, and then bring the bandage over one shoulder to keep it from slipping down around the trunk.

31

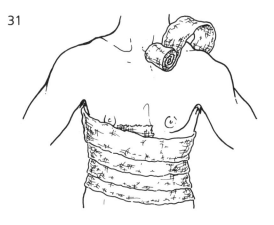

Take alternate turns around the trunk, over the shoulder, around the trunk, and so on.

32

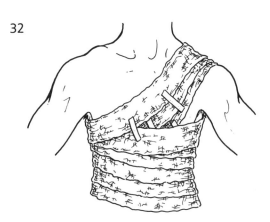

Stabilize the final dressing with strips of tape. It is usually possible to avoid taping the skin.

Such clumsy, large dressings can often be avoided by the use of Flexknit, underwear, and commercially available binders.

33

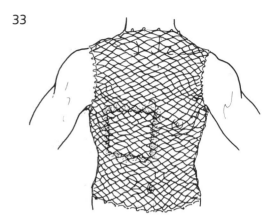

Flexknit gauze tubing can be fashioned into a vest by cutting two armholes.

Breast and Axilla

A bra provides the best dressing support for the breast. No tape is needed; simply position the dressing inside the bra. A bra in combination with a Flexknit tube for the arm can also provide excellent support for an axillary dressing.

34

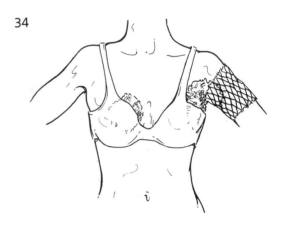

Abdomen

Commercial binders, easily washable and with Velcro closings, hold dressings well and are useful in cases requiring prolonged dressing care.

35

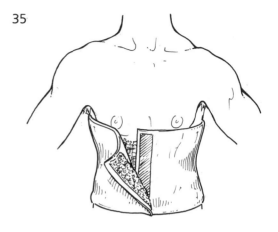

If a commercial binder is not available, one can be made of cotton piece goods, or a scultetus binder, an old-fashioned abdominal binder with many tails, can also serve as an inexpensive and effective method of holding a dressing. It tolerates laundering very well and can be reused for many months. When the tails are fastened with large safety pins, the scultetus binder will stay in place all day, even during considerable activity.

36

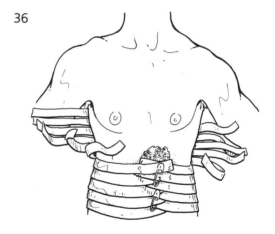

Abdominal dressings can often be held with panties or jockey-type shorts. One or two safety pins will hold the bandage in place; a perineal pad of the new adhesive Maxipad type can be used.

37

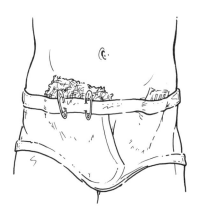

Perineum

The perineum is best dressed with sanitary napkins supported by a sanitary belt. Disposable adult diapers, sold under various trade names, also make excellent perineal dressings.

38

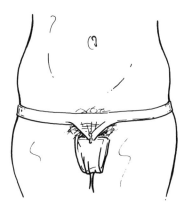

20 · *Surgical Infections and Antibiotic Usage*

BYRON BURLINGHAM, Ph.D.

The family physician is often faced with a wound contaminated by virulent opportunistic microbes in a patient with compromised defense mechanisms. In such cases, the doctor must cleanse the wound, control sources of contamination, enhance the patient's resistance, and administer antibiotics when indicated.

The incidence of surgical infections varies with the site and nature of the trauma. With massive contamination and tissue damage, incidence will be very high. Careful antisepsis, gentle technique, and proper postoperative care will reduce the incidence of infection in elective office procedures. Causes of wound infection other than surgical intervention may include contamination during induction of anesthesia, lowered host resistance, inadequate debridement, retained foreign bodies, continuing contamination, and nosocomial sources.

MECHANICS OF SURGICAL INFECTION

The patient's first defense against infection, an unbroken epithelium, is necessarily assaulted by a surgical procedure and interrupted by trauma, tumor, or inflammation. The outcome of a host-parasite interaction resulting in wound infection is defined by the Altemeir equation:

$$\text{Severity of wound infection or probability of wound infection} = \frac{\text{Number of inoculated} \times \text{Virulence of the organism}}{\text{Host defense mechanism}}$$

Of the variables, virulence of the organism cannot be altered by the family physician performing office surgery; it is determined by the genetics of the particular organism. The number

of organisms inoculated into the wound can be altered by asepsis and surgical technique, to some extent, as surgical pioneers such as Lister and Halsted demonstrated. Properly used, antibiotic prophylaxis is a pharmacological adjunct which acts in the extracellular space to reduce the inoculum. The host's defense mechanisms are greatly affected by the insults and stresses that occur before, during, and after surgery, such as instrumentation of the urinary tract, tissue trauma, and contamination of the wound

Table 1   Generalized Incidence of Clinical Infections in Surgical Patients

	Incidence Studies		Collective Summary of Antibiotic Prophylaxis[c]	
	NRC-USPHS[a]	Foothills[b]	Placebo	Antibiotic
Clean procedures	5.1%	1.5%	6.7%	3.2%
Clean-contaminated	10.8%	7.7%	26.3%	7.5%
Contaminated wounds	21.9%	15.2%	27.2%	12.6%
High risk, contaminated wounds		40.0%		
TOTAL	7.4%	4.7%		
Nosocomial infections (Surgical service)	4.9%			

[a]15,613 wounds, prospective study in 5 U.S. university centers; 1960–1963. Howard JM, et al. 1964. Ann Surg 160 (Suppl): 1.

[b]62,939 wounds, prospective study in Foothills Hospital, Calgary; 1967–1977. Cruse PJE, R Foord, 1980. Surg Clin. N.A. *66*:27.

[c]Data derived from tables comparing results of twenty-four critically evaluated reports. Chodak GW, ME Plaut, 1977. Arch Surg *112*:326; and Hirschmann JV, TS Inui, 1980. Rev Inf Dis. *2*:1.

[d]Bennett JV, PS Brachman, 1979. C13 in Hospital Infections, Bennett JV, PS Brachman, eds. Little, Brown & Company, Boston.

or the dressing, and by concomitant illness. Trauma, whether surgical or accidental, and the physiological response to it inevitably increase the patient's susceptibility to infection.

INDICATIONS OF INFECTION

An infection may be local or systemic. The patient's response will be directly related to the virulence of the organism; pyogenic organisms are likely to stimulate a dramatic response, whereas the nonpyogenic organisms, which are less virulent, will produce subtler and more ambiguous signs of infection. The partially or inadequately treated patient may also demonstrate milder response to infection. Focal infection is recognized by the classic signs of tumor, calor, rubor, and dolor. The more compromised the patient, the less dramatic will be the response to infection, and a severely compromised patient may have overwhelming sepsis with no symptoms whatsoever.

The normally reactive patient with acute infection typically has a modest fever, elevated white count with increased neutrophils, shift to the left in the Arneth count, elevated erythrocyte sedimentation rate, and elevated serum enzymes in association with the local site. In early infection by some virulent gram-positive bacteria, the circulating neutrophils will first be diminished and subsequently will rebound to very high numbers. In gram-negative sepsis, there may be a depressed or modestly elevated neutrophil count, with increased lymphocyte count. Chronic infections usually yield the same findings. Patients who have been treated with glucocorticosteroids or immunosuppressants will have a reduced or absent response to an invading pathogen. Late in overwhelming sepsis, the host's response may also be markedly reduced.

SPECIMEN COLLECTION

When infection is suspected, specimens should be collected either locally, if symptoms are localized, or systemically, if bacteremia or septicemia is suspected. Specimens may be taken from a wound, an abscess, a sinus tract, mucous membranes, or the respiratory tract; material for culture may be blood, cerebrospinal fluid, urine, or other secretions.

Accuracy of the laboratory findings will be limited by the competence of the person taking the specimen and by the procedures used for storage and transport. The specimen must come from infected tissue and must contain viable organisms for the pathogen to be identified. Specimens should be taken before antibiotic therapy is begun, or before it is changed, in the event of inadequate response to an antibiotic. Specimen containers should be sterile and free of any nonviable but potentially stainable organisms that might provide misleading results; they should also be leakproof to avoid contamination.

Unless proper aseptic technique is used, the normal flora of the epithelial surfaces can easily be introduced into a specimen. Before a venepuncture or biopsy, the skin should first be cleansed with 70% alcohol, followed by concentric application of 2% tincture of iodine or other idophor around the site. The antiseptic solution must remain in contact with the skin for *at least one minute* to be effective. The site should be touched or palpated only by a similarly disinfected or sterile-gloved finger.

Speedy transport and processing of specimens will increase the reliability of laboratory data. In general, microbes thrive in moist, warm, neutral-pH environments and do not survive desiccation, cold, and hostile pH. Pathogens in storage can often be overgrown by organisms from the normal flora before cultures can be made. Nearly all pathogenic and opportunistic microbes are anaerobes or facultative anaerobes; therefore, an anaerobic transport system is essential. Various gaseous mixtures can exclude oxygen from a specimen container; a transport medium containing resazurin as the indicator is best. When proper anaerobiosis is present, the resazurin remains colorless; if the transport medium is colored, however, the transport system should be discarded because it will be lethal to the sensitive anaerobes. Several commercial collection and transport systems containing a reducing gas generator and catalyst to scavenge any introduced oxygen are now available. When confronted with an unusual case, consult the laboratorian for special collection and transport materials.

Wound Culture

Material to be cultured from a wound ideally is aspirated with a sterile syringe rather than swabbed. Use of the swab should be limited to the skin and mucous membranes, and swabbed specimens should never be submitted when curettings, biopsy material, or surgically removed fluid or tissue are available. Before a direct aspirate is taken from an infected site, the contaminated superficial exudate or coagulum must first be removed; material for culture may then be drawn from the distal border of the active granulation tissue. Two specimens should be taken, with one being placed in anaerobic transport and the other in aerobic transport broth. Irrigation of the site with sterile, bacteriostat-free saline may yield sufficient material for the laboratory. Tissue from the wall of a lesion and from multiple sites will yield the most satisfactory results. Previously unopened and undrained abscesses will yield microorga-

nisms, provided the pus has been properly collected and transported. So-called sterile pus can usually be explained by careless collection of the specimen, improper transport of the specimen, or ineptness in the laboratory.

When a surgical wound is being closed, smears taken at the time of closure for quantitative biology can provide valuable prognostic information about the risk of sepsis. Gram's stain processing can provide quantitative data within 15 to 30 min of receipt of the specimen in the laboratory. If more than 10^5 colony-forming units are present per gram of material submitted, the risk of wound sepsis will be significantly increased.

Blood Culture

Patients without localized symptoms but with indications of infection are likely to have bacteremia. Repeated systematic blood cultures should be carried out when there is a sudden relative increase in the patient's pulse rate and temperature, a change in the sensorium, or onset of chills or prostration. Because most bacteremias are intermittent, collection of blood for culture should be made intermittently during a 24-hr period. But even within the constraints of an office practice, a single blood culture can be obtained readily. It is useful; a single blood culture will be positive about 80% of the time, and three blood cultures within 24 hr will indicate with nearly 100% accuracy any clinically significant bacteremias. A very large sample of blood taken at one time and divided does not constitute multiple cultures. Blood samples may be contaminated by normal skin flora, but isolation of the same organisms from multiple blood cultures obtained by separate venepunctures lends credence to the laboratory findings.

Intra-abdominal Infection

Anaerobes are involved in 85% of intra-abdominal infections, 50 to 100% of liver abscesses, and at least 90% of pelvic and pararectal abscesses. If the pathogens are to be isolated, several milliliters of pus obtained at paracentesis or culpocentesis or a sizable mass of tissue (2 to 3 mm) must be collected and properly transported under anaerobic conditions. Air bubbles must be expelled from a syringe, if the specimen is to be transported therein, and the needle should be plugged with a sterile rubber stopper. Most anaerobic infections are of a mixed type and may be quite confusing to interpret.

Cerebrospinal Fluid

Stringent aseptic technique is required for both patient and specimen in collection of cerebrospinal fluid for culture. Preparation of the site with tincture of iodine or an iodophor is necessary to avoid contamination by normal skin flora. The tubes must be sterile and free of any stainable material. Spinal fluid specimens must be transported to the laboratory quite rapidly and examined promptly since many of the organisms will not survive storage. In most cases of bacterial meningitis, more than 10^5 bacteria are present per milliliter of specimen material; these can be detected by direct smear and stain. Anaerobic bacteria, present in 90% of brain abscesses, can be detected by anaerobic culture.

Respiratory Tract Cultures

About 16% of surgical patients develop respiratory tract infections during their hospital stay. With the present trend to shorter postoperative stays, patients with such infections are often seen in the family physician's office. Culture of material from the upper respiratory tract is easy to perform but is usually nonproductive because normal individuals frequently support potentially pathogenic or opportunistic microbes and rich microflora in the upper tract. Sputum collected in the office is usually heavily contaminated with such flora, and such specimens will be overgrown by this flora if they are not promptly delivered to the laboratory. Routine sputum culture is not recommended for diagnosis of acute bacterial pneumonitis. Correlation between results of parallel cultures of tracheal aspirates and sputum cultures is poor, and there is currently no satisfactory means of isolating bacterial pathogens from expectorated sputum. Anaerobic culture of sputum is not useful and should be avoided.

Organisms comprising the normal microflora of the upper respiratory tract become pathogens when they colonize the lower tract. Even though samples from the lower tract are difficult to obtain, specimens properly collected from it can yield rewarding information. Percutaneous transtracheal aspiration is the best method. This relatively harmless, rapidly performed procedure, done under local anesthesia, is especially useful in patients who cannot raise sputum or in those suspected of having anaerobic pleuropulmonary infection. Nasotracheal or bronchial washes or aspirates may also be satisfactory. Pulmonary infection may also occasionally be diagnosed by percutaneous transthoracic needle biopsy, needle aspiration, thoracentesis, or open lung biopsy.

Urine Specimens

Urinary tract infections are the most common type of infection seen in the hospital and the doctor's office. About 14% of surgical patients develop significant bacteriuria during their hospital stay. Collection of urine specimens is not a task for the least experienced office aide; it should be performed under adequate supervision or by someone who understands the proper technique.

For male patients, a clean-catch midstream specimen is reliable for diagnosis, provided the patient is circumcised or has been properly prepared by retraction of the foreskin and cleansing of the glans. Catheterized specimens are usually procured only if a urologic procedure is being performed concurrently. When a specimen is obtained by catheterization, there should be a free flow of urine at the time of collection, and the specimen must come directly from the catheter rather than from the collection bag, which is usually contaminated.

Thorough perineal preparation is required for proper collection of a voided specimen from a female patient. The specimen should be checked at once for squamous epithelial cells; if these are seen, the specimen has been improperly collected, and another must be obtained. In female patients, when preparation has been correct, diagnosis of infection from a urine specimen is reliable about 80% of the time.

Specimens from children are best collected by suprapubic aspiration. All urine specimens except for carefully collected suprapubic aspirates contain urethral flora, which will overgrow the pathogens, yielding misleading results, unless the urine specimen is rapidly chilled to 4 to 5 degrees C and transported immediately to the laboratory.

In urine cultures, a count of 10^5 or more bacteria per milliliter is valid evidence for active infection as opposed to contamination. A direct Gram's stain will show at least two bacteria in each oil immersion (1,000X) field at 10^5 bacteria per milliliter. Turbidity appears in the urine at 10^7 bacteria per milliliter and is prominent at 10^8 to 10^9. Generally speaking, gram-positive organisms in urine are skin contaminants, whereas gram-negative organisms are likely true potential pathogens.

MICROBIOLOGIC STUDIES

Routine microbiologic tests include direct stain, culture and identification, susceptibility testing (antibiograms), and, when required, minimum inhibitory concentration (MIC). Direct staining, a frequently overlooked technique, is inexpensive, quick, and easily done in the office. When localizing symptoms occur, the microorganism can usually be seen in a direct stain. Direct staining gives information about the groups of organisms present, an estimate of their relative and absolute concentrations, and indications as to which are merely contaminants and which are the true pathogens. In an acute infection, the Gram's stain alone will supply the family physician with information directing him or her to the most appropriate antibiotic. Most chronic or smoldering infections can await laboratory test results.

Susceptibility testing is indicated when clinically significant organisms of unpredictable susceptibility (staphylococci, enterobacteriaceae, pseudomonas) are isolated from normally sterile sites. Susceptibility testing is well standardized and reliable for aerobes and facultative anaerobes. Testing for obligate anaerobes is not routinely done; these organisms are genetically stable and predictable, their slow growth delays testing, and they are usually involved in polymicrobic infection.

The serological assay is frequently overlooked, but in many chronic infections acute and convalescent sera can be very informative. The physician who expects an illness to be acute and quickly responsive may not think of collecting a specimen at the onset of the illness. However, in about one-third of cases where response is not immediate, further laboratory studies are called for; thus, the physician would be wise to draw a few milliliters of clotted blood for storage in the refrigerator in case serological tests are needed. After the infection has cleared, the specimen may be discarded.

ANTIMICROBIAL THERAPY

Choice of an appropriate antimicrobial agent for an infection involves several considerations:

- Identification of the organism, or a reasonable guess about its identity, based on clinical information;

- Accurate information about the sensitivity of the organism;

- Nature of the underlying pathologic process and its natural history;

- Immune status of the host;

- Pharmacologic properties of the drugs being considered and route of administration;

- Clinical history, including previous adverse reactions, age of the patient, genetic or metabolic abnormalities, presence or absence of pregnancy, hepatic and renal function, and route of infection.

Antibiograms (MIC) will indicate the most suitable antibiotic for a particular pathogen. In general, the oldest effective drug with the lowest toxicity in the specific patient is the best choice. When no pathogen can be isolated, the physician must choose empirically the drug to be used. The tendency seems to have been to use multiple drugs with the broadest possible and overlapping spectra, but a better strategy would be to select one antimicrobial agent, on the basis of the laboratory data and clinical picture. This approach has significant benefits for the patient; combining antimicrobial drugs is risky, expensive, and usually of little benefit. Only a few justifications exist for combining antimicrobials:

- Prevention of the emergence of resistant organisms (documented as effective only in tuberculosis);

- Polymicrobial infections—if a broad spectrum of organisms is involved, as in brain abscesses or in intraperitoneal or pelvic infections by mixed bowel flora, combining antimicrobials may be helpful;

- Initial therapy in neutropenic patients while awaiting results of cultures—in this instance it is reasonable to begin broad-spectrum coverage, usually with nafcillin or carbenicillin in combination with gentamicin or tobramycin, until the pathogen is identified;

- Decreasing toxicity of a combination to the host by decreasing the dose of each drug, with high selective toxicity remaining for the infecting organism; this has been established only for triple sulfa, in which instance, because of the partial solubilities of the drugs, crystalluria and calculi are reduced;

- Synergism between two agents, rarely demonstrated in vivo—for example, a penicillin and aminoglycoside for enterococcal endocarditis, a penicillinase-resistant penicillin with an aminoglycoside for massive pseudomonas infection, amphotericin B with 5-fluorocytosine against fungi, and trimethoprim and sulfamethoxazole for resistant salmonella, shigella, or *Hemophilus influenzae.*

A patient infected with a gram-positive organism who fails to respond within 24 hr to the antibiotic of choice as determined by an antibiogram or MIC, or a patient with a gram-negative organism who fails to respond to the antibiotic within 72 hr should have blood levels of the antibiotic measured. Failure to respond to an antibiotic after proper in vitro sensitivity testing is attributable to less than therapeutic levels of the drug in blood or tissue, because of insufficient doses, poor absorption, or a metabolic idiosyncracy in the patient. The physician must determine the cause and compensate for it by increasing the dose or changing the antibiotic.

A patient may not improve with antibiotic therapy if his or her defense mechanisms are impaired. A white blood cell count and response and determination of the number of lymphocytes and platelets are helpful in evaluation of the patient's defense mechanism. A patient with diminished ability to respond to appropriate antibiotic therapy may require transfusions of white cells or infusion of specific immunoglobulins and should be hospitalized.

Prophylaxis

One-fourth to one-half of all antimicrobial drugs given on surgical services are for prevention rather than treatment of infection. The proper role of antimicrobial prophylaxis has been very controversial and the effect is documented in Table 1. The benefits increase as the risks of infection increase. Some question whether the overall benefit in clean procedures merits use. Nearly all studies indicate that patients with clean-contaminated and contaminated procedures are benefitted. With increasing contamination of the wound, the antibiotic is no longer prophylactic, but part of a therapeutic regimen. Theoretically, the role of antibiotic prophylaxis should be greater in the compromised patient, but this has not been evaluated. Similarly, many office procedures are properly covered with prophylactic antibacterial drugs. Antibiotic prophylaxis, *properly used* in a surgical office practice, calls for an appropriate broad-spectrum antibiotic, usually given parenterally, to achieve a bactericidal concentration in the tissue during the operative procedure. If surgery is delayed or prolonged, a second dose may be advisable. Continuing antibiotic prophylaxis longer than 24 hr increases the patient's risk of infection.

Complications of Antimicrobial Therapy

Complications of antimicrobial therapy fall into three categories: (1) organ toxicity and hypersensitivity, (2) superinfection, and (3) nosocomial impact. As bacteria have acquired genetic resistance to antibiotic drugs, antimicrobials of less selective toxicity have had to be used. These drugs attack metabolic pathways in both bacteria and host, with direct toxicity for particular organs or tissues. Many antimicrobials are charged molecules that bind to human proteins, thus becoming haptenic antigens or allergens that stimulate a humoral or cell-mediated response, or both. Subsequent or continued exposure may bring about a hypersensitivity reaction with serious sequelae or even fatality.

It is not true that the only good bacterium is a dead bacterium. The normal bacterial flora of the epithelium is beneficial and protective, and long-term broad-spectrum shotgun antibiotic therapy may devastate the normal flora, allowing new flora to grow to overwhelming numbers; the result is superinfection. This is especially a risk to the more compromised patient.

Infections by opportunistic bacteria and fungi have recently increased, and natural and therapeutic immunosuppression has served to activate latent viruses, especially the herpes group (varicella, herpes simplex and zoster, cytomegalovirus, and Epstein-Barr). Diminished host resistance is the underlying condition that permits such organisms to flourish, and the physician cannot always bolster this resistance. Termination of the drug therapy may be a temporary solution, but the pathologic condition that originally necessitated the treatment will not have been eliminated.

Because an antibiotic always applies selective pressure for genetic resistance in the normal flora, genes for resistance may be acquired and shared among the normal flora, opportunists, and invading pathogens. Obviously, hospital flora will be affected by this circumstance; in some species, virulence genes have become linked with genes for antibiotic resistance. Antimicrobial agents, properly applied, are vital to control infection in individual patients, but widespread, indiscriminate use of such drugs has a broad impact on the environment. Each time a physician prescribes an antibiotic, he or she must weigh the benefits to the individual patient against the risk to the same patient and to others in the same environment.

21 · *Office Surgery of the Breast*

WALTER J. PORIES, M.D.

Surgical problems of the breast are common, and many of them can be handled in the physician's office. Office surgery saves delay and cost and, most important, helps allay patients' fears and promotes early diagnosis of cancer.

Several important points need to be made. First, because women with breast problems are often frightened and the breast is a sensitive organ, premedication with a tranquilizer such as 5 mg of diazepam or a similar agent is helpful. Liberally infiltrate the local anesthetic agent and allow at least 10 min by the clock to produce adequate anesthesia.

Second, make incisions circular, in line with the areola, or in the fold under the breast. Circumareolar incisions are best and leave almost invisible scars. Spoke-of-a-wheel incisions radiating outward from the nipple and cruciate incisions leave ugly scars and should be avoided.

1

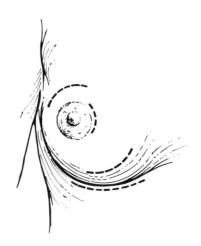

Third, because some breasts have a liberal blood supply, brisk bleeding can be encountered during a procedure in mammary tissue. Such hemorrhage may be difficult to control because the bleeding vessels often retract into the fat. Be prepared to handle such a situation, clamping and controlling each vessel as it comes into view and having available some large stout needles, such as the large Mayos with swaged-on 2-0 Dexon or Vicryl for hemostatic sutures.

Fourth, after the surgery, the wound should be dry. If there is even limited ooze, place a drain so blood can escape, or else a huge hematoma may form. We have seen these extend around the chest, down the abdomen, and even onto the thighs.

Finally, the best dressing for the breast is one or two thicknesses of 4 × 4s tucked without tape into the patient's bra. Kotex or Maxipads cut to the appropriate size make excellent absorbent and inexpensive dressings if multiple changes are expected.

2

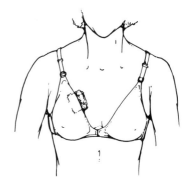

ASPIRATION OF BREAST MASSES

Most breast masses are not cancerous; many are cysts. If the mass is about 1 cm or larger, aspiration is a useful, inexpensive, immediate, and safe test to tell whether the lesion is cystic or solid.

Extend the patient's arm on an arm board or, better, place it under her head.

3

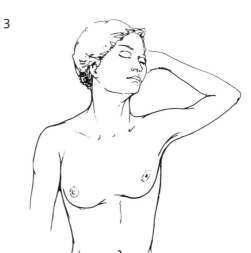

Gently paint the breast with Betadine.

4

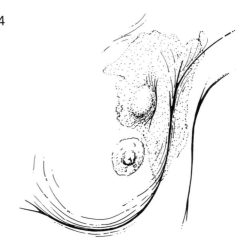

Anesthesia is not normally needed. Hold the mass between two fingers to fix it to the chest wall and push a #18 or #19 needle attached to a 10-ml syringe into the center of the lump. Aspiration usually produces a cloudy yellow or greenish fluid. If the first attempt is unsuccessful, several other tries can be made without pain to the patient if the needle is not withdrawn from the skin on each pass.

5

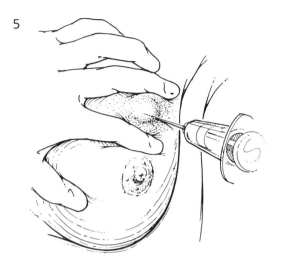

The aspirate, whether the aspiration is successful or dry, should be sprayed onto a slide, fixed with fixative, and sent for cytologic examination.

6

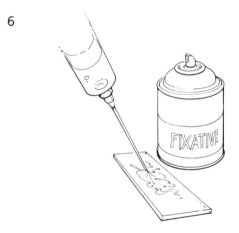

Often, enough cells are obtained from a dry aspirate to make a diagnosis of breast cancer. *If the aspiration is not successful or if the lesion does not totally disappear, the lesion must be considered to have a high probability of cancer.* Patients with such lesions should be referred promptly for mammography and surgical consultation.

Re-examine the patient in a month. It is most unusual for a cyst to recur; if the mass is again present on the follow-up examination, promptly arrange for mammography and excision.

NEEDLE BIOPSY

Needle biopsy with a disposable Tru-cut needle is a valuable technique for confirming the diagnosis of cancer in large neglected lesions or suspected recurrences.

7

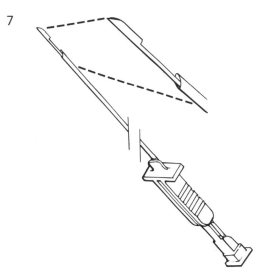

Anesthetize a small area over the center of the tumor, and make a small (3 to 4 mm) incision with the point of a #11 or #15 blade to let the Tru-cut needle enter if the lesion has not ulcerated through the skin. If the tumor tissue is exposed, no anesthesia is necessary.

Insert the tip of the closed Tru-cut needle into the tumor to a distance of 2 to 3 mm.

8

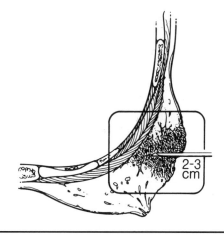

2-3 cm

Advance the inner shaft of the needle deeply into the tumor. Advance the outer hub, which serves as a circular blade, over the inner shaft to cut a core of the tumor.

9

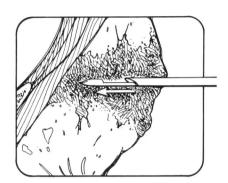

The core should be a suitable specimen, 1 × 5 to 10 mm in size. It is usually white or grey and quite firm. If a suitable core has not been obtained, make another pass. Place the specimen in formalin and send it for pathologic examination.

10

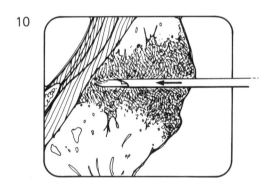

11

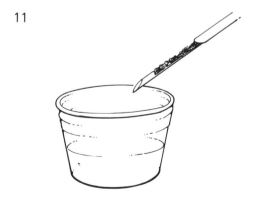

DISCHARGES FROM THE NIPPLE

Nipple discharges are common and are not often malignant. They are occasionally of short duration and, in such instances, are probably due to hormonal imbalances; if they last more than one or two months, however, they are probably associated with an intraductal papilloma or cystic disease of the breast.

The initial step of the investigation should be a cytologic examination of the discharge. Gently squeeze the breast; the patient usually knows the best site to press. Smear the material on a slide, fix it, and send it for pathologic examination. Bloody discharges are more worrisome than those without blood, but in women over 40, we also recommend that a mammogram be done.

12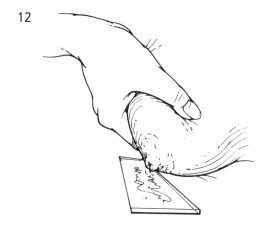

If the discharge persists, refer the patient to have the offending duct excised, because the natural history of papillomas is for continuing growth and increasing discharge. Because they are sometimes voluminous, nipple discharges can be an embarrassing problem.

BREAST BIOPSY

Small superficial breast lesions can be excised in the office, but we urge a review of the points noted at the beginning of this chapter before undertaking such a procedure.

Particularly suitable for office surgery are the mobile and discrete fibroadenomas, often called "breast mice" because of their apparent mobility under the skin. Small superficial areas of coalesced and suspicious cystic disease or individual small firm masses near the surface of the breast also lend themselves to excision under local anesthesia. The patient is also a part of the equation, however; nervous, frightened patients may not tolerate hospital biopsies well.

Outline the incision with a ballpoint pen before infiltrating any anesthetic because the local anesthetic is likely to obliterate the outlines of the lesion. Inject about 20 to 30 ml of 1% lidocaine with epinephrine around *and below* the lesion.

13

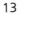
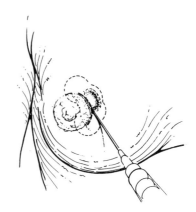

To make the incision most easily, push down firmly around the areola to tighten and stabilize the skin for the incision. Carry the incision through the dermis until the subareolar plexus of vessels is identified.

14

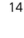
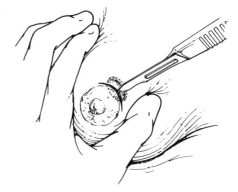

Cauterize the subareolar plexus for hemostasis.

15

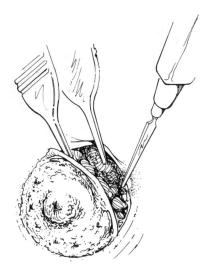

Push a stout Mayo needle with a 2-0 swaged-on suture through the mass twice. The suture serves as a convenient handle for the specimen during the excision with cautery.

16

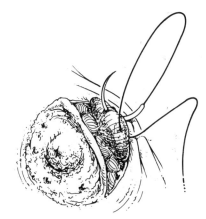

Cauterize or clamp and tie each vessel as it appears. When arteries and veins of the breast retract into the breast tissue or the fat, they can be most difficult to manage.

17

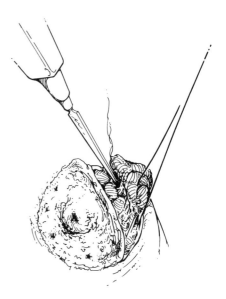

The gross appearance of the lesion usually indicates its pathology. Circumscribed lesions with a well-demarcated capsule are usually benign. If the material is white, hard, and gritty, the lesion is probably cancerous; if the tissue is grey and uniform with fine whorls, the lesion is probably a fibroadenoma; and if there are multiple small pockets of fluid, the problem is most likely fibrocystic disease. It is essential, of course, that this initial impression be confirmed by a formal pathologic examination.

Close the incision using a running subcuticular suture of 4-0 Vicryl or Dexon.

18

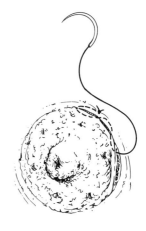

A 1/2-in Steri-strip dressing is usually the only dressing needed.

19

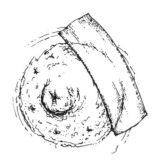

If the field is not absolutely dry at the end of the excision, insert a small drain, such as a 1/4-in Penrose. Partially close the incision. Suture the drain in place with a small stitch, and mark it well with a sterile safety pin.

20

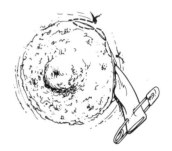

DRAINAGE OF BREAST ABSCESSES

Breast abscesses are often insidious and may therefore be neglected too long. Consider every apparent case of mastitis with fever and a tender red breast an abscess until proven otherwise by a negative aspiration. Fluctuance, one of the signs that an abscess is ripe, may never appear in the breast because there is no fascial envelope compressing the pus. A breast abscess is therefore diagnosed not so much by physical examination as by needle aspiration. Perform this test when the patient is first seen with an inflamed breast, and repeat it if the infection does not rapidly clear with antibiotics. If pus is aspirated, promptly drain the breast to avoid the risks of extension of the infection and even destruction of the breast.

Infiltrate the tenderest area over the lesion with lidocaine and epinephrine. When the area has been anesthetized, introduce a #18 needle and a 10-ml syringe into the center of the inflammatory area and begin gentle aspiration. Withdraw only a minimal amount of pus. Keep the needle in place to help in finding the pocket of pus during incision and drainage.

21

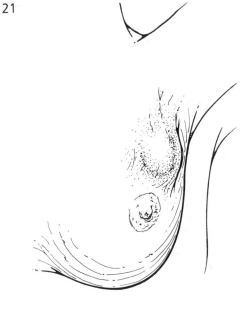

22

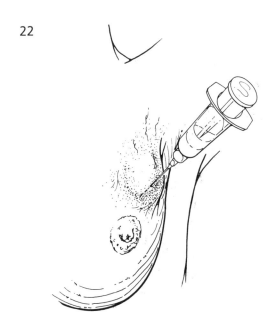

Incise the breast in a semicircular direction. The 23
knife hugs the needle closely during the incision
so that the pocket is not missed and so that
the inflammatory and highly vascular tissues
around the pus are avoided as much as possible.
False cuts into the surrounding phlegmon can
produce troublesome bleeding. Cruciate incisions are not necessary, cause delayed healing,
and leave ugly scars. Avoid them.

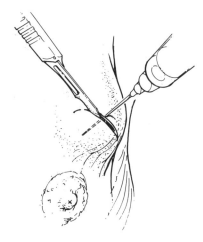

The incision need not be large, and it is not
necessary to explore the cavity with a finger or
a clamp to destroy any loculating septa. We
consider this a painful and unnecessary maneuver, which probably does more harm than good
by violating the walls of the abscess.

Insert a small Malecot catheter to ensure con- 24
tinued drainage.

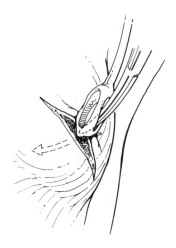

Culture and examine the material from the syringe with Gram's stain to guide the choice of appropriate antibiotics.

25

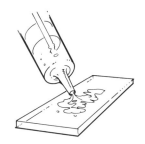

Leave the catheter in place until the drainage ceases or becomes minimal, usually about two to four weeks; breast abscesses heal slowly. Protect the patient with a broad-spectrum antibiotic for one week, and encourage her to stay at home and rest. Warm, moist compresses make the patient more comfortable, promote better drainage, and lead to faster resolution.

26

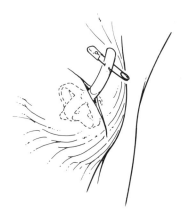

If the abscess does not subside promptly, a sinogram is advisable to determine whether good drainage has been achieved. Similarly, mammography can be of great help in assessing the progress of healing and in assuring that no serious underlying pathology, such as a malignancy, is missed.

22 · *Office Surgery of the Urinary Tract*

ED JANOSKO, M.D.

Urologic surgery is most appropriately performed by a trained urologist. However, circumstances may dictate otherwise. Three procedures can be performed by the trained family physician when a urologic surgeon may not be available: (1) catheterization of the obstructed urinary bladder, (2) circumcision, and (3) vasectomy.

CATHETERIZATION FOR URINARY RETENTION

Acute urinary retention is a common urological problem and an obvious emergency. The physician must relieve the retention by drainage of the bladder in the least traumatic and painful manner. This effort should be approached systematically, as shown.

1

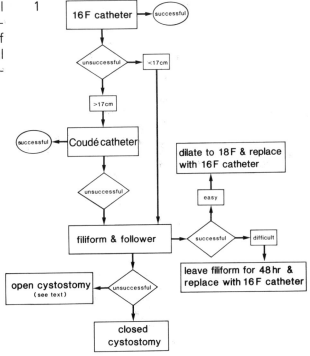

In the female, catheterization is rarely difficult; obstacles might be a retracted or hypospadiac meatus or marked meatal stenosis. When the patient is placed in the lithotomy position, catheterization with a #16 French catheter, with or without a catheter guide, should be easily accomplished.

In the male, the most common obstacles to easy catheterization are urethral stricture, prostatic disease (either benign or carcinomatous), or bladder-neck contracture following prostatectomy. If a #16 French catheter cannot be easily introduced into the bladder, all efforts to insert it should be stopped immediately, before urethral trauma occurs, and the physician must continue the diagnostic investigation.

The patient must be asked whether his urinary stream has been decreased and whether he has hesitance or voiding problems that suggest prostatism or urethral stricture. He should be asked about past history of urethral trauma, instrumentation, gonorrheal disease, or prostatectomy. The patient should then be examined to determine the degree of retention and the size of the bladder. Rectal examination should be performed to evaluate the size and consistency of the prostate gland. Next, the perineum is prepared with an antiseptic solution. A water-soluble jelly (Lubafax) or, if available, an anesthetic jelly (1% lignocaine, or Anestacon) is introduced into the urethra gently with a syringe. A #16 Foley catheter is then gently introduced. If the catheter cannot be passed beyond the first 17 cm, the problem is most likely a urethral stricture. If the obstruction lies beyond 17 cm, it is probably due to prostatism, carcinoma of the prostate, or bladder-neck contracture.

Figure 2 demonstrates the basic set of catheters that should be available in the physician's office.

2

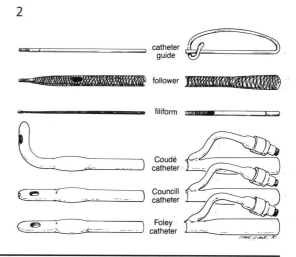

catheter guide

follower

filiform

Coudé catheter

Councill catheter

Foley catheter

If prostatism is suspected, one should try to pass a #16 French Coudé catheter, which will usually slip over the median lobe. If this fails, urethrography should be performed, but if facilities for it are not available, one must then proceed with the use of filiforms and followers.

3

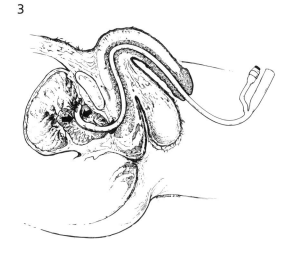

The filiform, in a size between #3 and #6 French, should be introduced slowly until resistance is met; it is then passed back and forth until it falls through the stricture and enters the bladder. If the filiform will not pass the stricture, it should be advanced as far as it will go and left in place; other filiforms should then be passed sequentially until one finally falls through the stricture into the bladder.

4

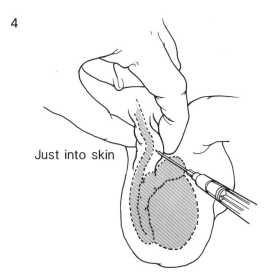

Just into skin

Once a filiform is in the bladder, the remaining filiforms are removed and the stricture is dilated gently, starting with a #8 French follower.

5

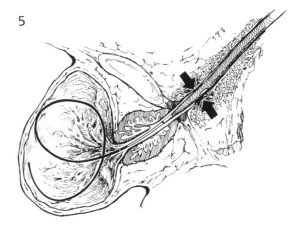

6

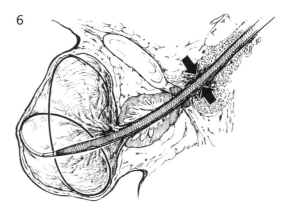

If the passage of either the filiform or the follower has been especially difficult, the follower should be taped in place to drain for 48 hr. During this interval, the stricture will soften and the urethra will mold around the follower. Later, after 48 hr, one should have no difficulty in introducing a catheter into the bladder.

7

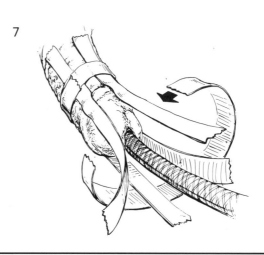

Often the stricture is easily dilated from #8 to #18 French by the filiform-and-follower technique, with progressively larger followers screwed onto the initial filiform. An ordinary catheter or a Councill catheter may then be placed in the bladder. The Councill catheter, placed over a catheter guide screwed onto the filiform and adequately lubricated, is gently passed into the bladder. The balloon is then inflated. The filiform and the catheter guide are then removed, leaving the Councill catheter in the bladder.

8

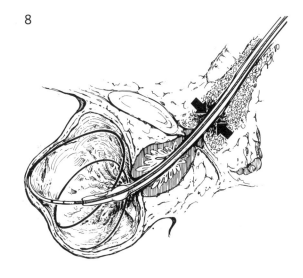

9

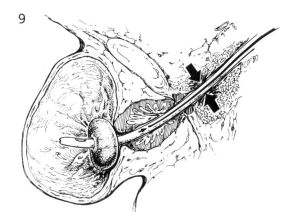

When neither a catheter nor filiform can be passed and bladder-neck contracture seems likely, a #20 French urethral sound should be gently inserted but never pushed forcibly. This maneuver is not usually successful, but with bladder-neck contracture the sound will sometimes pass over the lip of the contracture, after which a catheter can be molded on a catheter guide and passed.

It is imperative that sounds and catheter guides be inserted with great care because they can cause extensive damage. The most common sites of urethral perforation by these instruments are just proximal to a urethral stricture or just below the prostate. For difficult situations, or if the physician is not familiar with sounding, suprapubic cystostomy is strongly recommended.

10

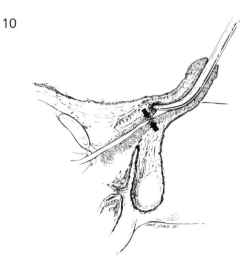

In the rare case of an impassable urethra, suprapubic cystostomy will certainly be called for. For placement of a catheter in this manner, the bladder is palpated just above the pubic ramus. The lower abdomen is prepared with an antiseptic solution, and lignocaine is infiltrated at a point approximately one-third of the distance between the pubic ramus and the umbilicus.

11

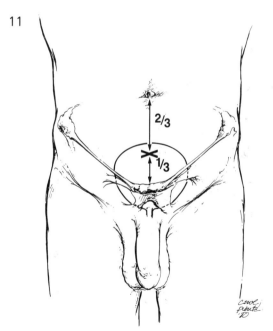

A Cystocath catheter is introduced through a trocar at a 60-degree angle toward the pubic tubercle and passed gently through the skin and rectus sheath into the bladder.

12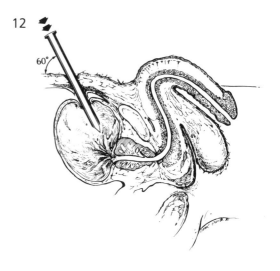

13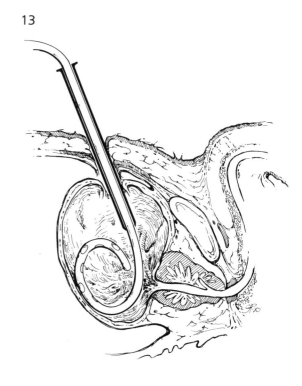

This catheter is secured in place and left indwelling, and a voiding cystourethrogram or retrograde urethrogram can later be performed unhurriedly to define the disease. Contraindications to the closed suprapubic technique are previous pelvic surgery, bladder carcinoma, or an impalpable or small bladder. In these cases, an open cystostomy is required.

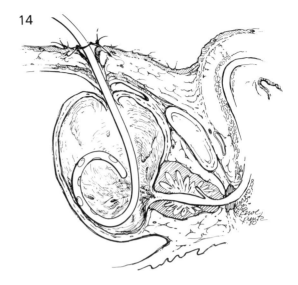

14

One may occasionally have to deal with severe phimosis or edema of the foreskin, from anasarca or localized infection. In such cases, a dorsal slit must be created to expose the glans and the meatus.

CIRCUMCISION

Circumcision is a common procedure, performed more often for religious or social purposes than for true medical indications. The medical indications for circumcision are phimosis, paraphimosis, balanitis, and posthitis not resolving with medical therapy.

Preparation

With the patient supine, the skin at the base of the penis is shaved of all hair. The entire genitalia, scrotum, and lower abdomen are prepped with an antiseptic solution and draped with a disposable towel with a central perforation.

Procedure

Using a 10-cc syringe filled with 1% lidocaine
and a 1-1/2-in 22-gauge needle, inject subcutaneously over the dorsal vein of the penopubic
junction, raising a skin wheal. On either side of
the dorsal vein, extend the needle subcutaneously to the tunica albuginea, which is felt as
a firm layer. Inject circumferentially close to the
tunica albuginea on either side. The needle is
then removed.

15

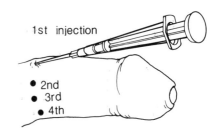

Place a 1/4-in Penrose drain around the penis
and clamp it firmly with a hemostat to obstruct
venous outflow. Refill the syringe with 5 cc of
1% lidocaine and inject 2 cc into both corpora
cavernosa just distal to the Penrose drain.

16

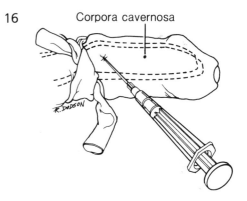

With the final 1 cc, infiltrate the frenulum subcutaneously. Wait 10 min for the anesthetic to
become effective, and then remove the Penrose
drain.

17

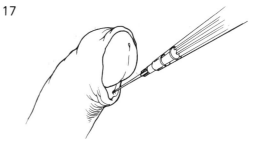

Grasp the foreskin in the 3 and 9 o'clock positions with hemostats and pull the foreskin over the glans penis. Place two straight hemostats in the 11 and 1 o'clock positions on the prepuce, and make an incision with the Mayo scissors at the 12 o'clock position to within 1 cm of the corona. Place two straight hemostats in the 5 and 7 o'clock positions to the base of the frenulum, and incise the prepuce with the Mayo scissors to the base of the frenulum in the 6 o'clock position. This leaves two wings of the prepuce, which are then placed on retraction. Using the Mayo scissors, cut the wings of the prepuce to within 1 cm of the corona.

18

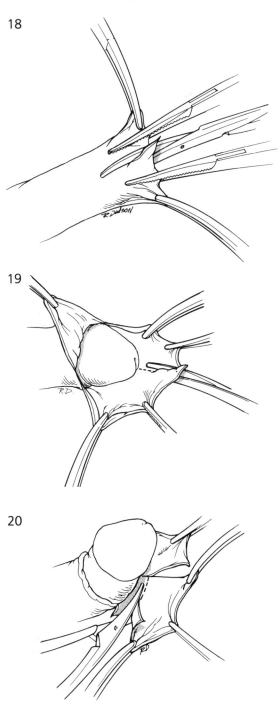

19

20

Fulgurate all bleeders with appropriate cautery, and ligate the large dorsal vein, if cut, with 3-0 plain catgut suture. Obtain complete hemostasis. The penile shaft skin is then sewn to the distal coronal skin with interrupted sutures of 4-0 chromic.

21

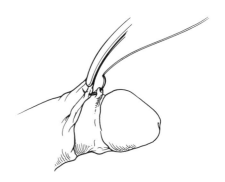

Vaseline gauze is placed on the incision site. The patient is then given an analgesic to take every 4 hr for pain if needed. No drug will prevent erections, so none should be given for this purpose. The patient is then asked the following day to soak in a warm tub of water and remove the Vaseline gauze. From then on, he is to replace the gauze daily around the incision site. The patient is seen two weeks later, and intercourse is usually allowed to resume in three to four weeks.

22

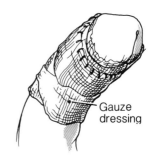

Gauze dressing

VASECTOMY

Bilateral partial vasectomy is a relatively uncomplicated procedure that produces sterility by interrupting the vas deferens. The patient as well as his wife, if he is married, should be appropriately counseled about the permanence of the procedure and possible recanalization and failure. Although reversible vasectomy has been popular and successful, no one can guarantee this result for a particular patient. There is no contraindication to vasectomy except an active epididymitis.

23a

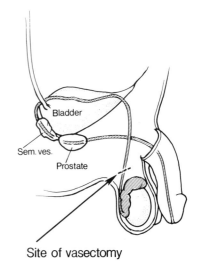

Bladder

Sem. ves.

Prostate

Site of vasectomy

Preparation

The patient is instructed to shave his scrotal skin and shower with a pHisoHex or Betadine solution just prior to the office visit. For the procedure, he is placed in the dorsal lithotomy position. The genitalia are then prepped with a warm antiseptic solution.

Procedure

With the left hand, grasp the vas between the thumb and forefinger, and rotate the vas until it is just below the skin level. Using a 10-cc syringe and a 25-gauge needle, inject the overlying scrotal skin and the dartos muscle lateral to each side of the vas with 3 to 4 cc of 1% lidocaine with epinephrine.

23b

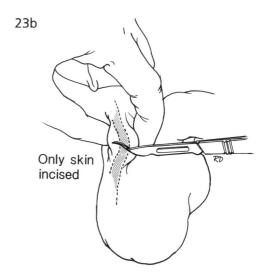

Only skin
incised

Incise the skin for 1 cm over the vas with a #15 scalpel blade.

24

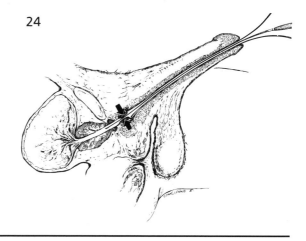

Separate the underlying dartos fascia with the hemostat.

25

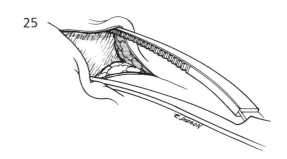

Using the Allis clamp, grasp the vas within its confines, and gently place this on traction. Inject 2 cc more of lidocaine within the fascial sheath overlying the vas proximally and ventrally. Use the scalpel to dissect the overlying fascial layers away from the underlying vas. When the vas is exposed anteriorly, use a towel clamp and place this around the vas, separating it from the vasal artery.

26a

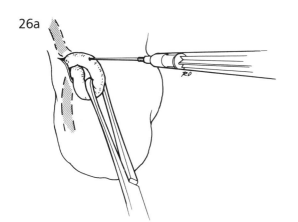

26b

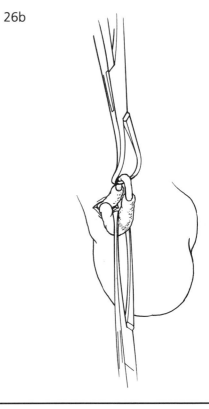

Remove the Allis clamp and place it distally, and with another towel clamp dissect the vas away from the fascial layers.

Grasp the vas with a pickup, cut the vas distally, and fulgurate its lumen.

27

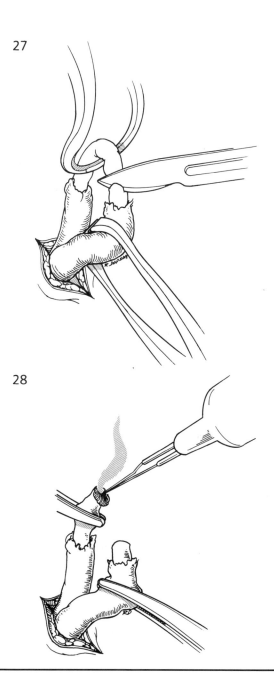

28

Let that end of the vas retract, and remove approximately 1 cm of the remaining vas and fulgurate the proximal lumen. Close the fascia over the retracted vas with a figure-eight suture of 4-0 chromic, and lightly tie the ends of this suture around the distal vas to occlude the space between the fascia and the proximal vas. The vas is then allowed to retract back into the scrotum, and the skin and dartos are closed with a single layer with two to three sutures of 4-0 chromic. A similar procedure is performed on the opposite side.

29

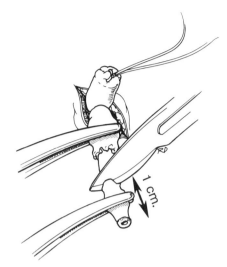

30

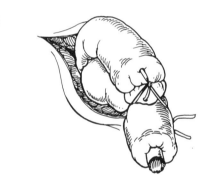

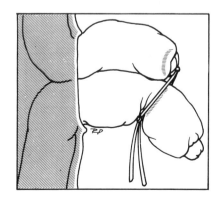

Instructions

The patient is sent home with an athletic supporter with gauze over the incision. He is instructed to place an ice pack on the scrotum for 6 hr following the operation and to remain quiet, either sitting or at bedrest for that evening. The following day, he is allowed to ambulate freely but not to strain, and by 48 hr activity is limited only by the patient's discomfort.

A mild analgesic is given for pain, and he is allowed to take a shower the following day. Sex is prohibited for one week, and normal sexual relations are allowed to resume after that. **The patient must be warned that he is not sterile at this time.** A semen analysis is obtained at six weeks. If this shows no evidence of any sperm, another one is repeated at eight weeks, and if this too is negative, the patient is discharged. If any sperm are present in the semen, follow-up semen analyses are obtained at two-week intervals until no sperm are left. If after three months the patient has had more than twenty ejaculations and there are still sperm left in the semen, one must consider failure and recanalization of the vas, and revasectomy must be performed. Minor complications such as bleeding from the skin edges, mild epididymitis from obstruction, or sperm granuloma can usually be handled conservatively with skin compression, anti-inflammatory agents, and antibiotics.

23 · *Treatment of Pilonidal Sinus*

WALTER J. PORIES, M.D.

Pilonidal sinuses are common lesions at the base of the spine and are frequently the site of infection in young patients, especially those who are hirsute. Various surgical procedures have been described for this condition, but none produces better results than the simple approaches described in this chapter.

PREVENTION

Most problems with pilonidal sinuses can be easily prevented. If a pilonidal pit, or sinus, is discovered during a physical examination, advise the patient to keep the area shaved and to have someone withdraw the curious long strands of hair from the cavity with a fine pair of tweezers. The hair is never attached and, although there are many opinions, no one knows how the hair gets there.

1

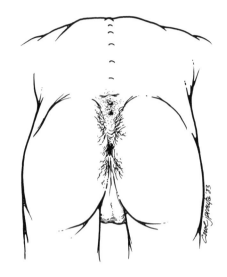

2

3

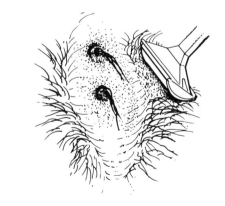

ACUTE PILONIDAL ABSCESS

If there is an abscess, shave the area and paint it with Betadine. Liberally infiltrate the tenderest area with lidocaine and epinephrine. Determining the site of greatest tenderness helps in locating the area where the pus is most easily drained.

4

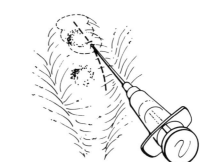

Make a small incision (about 1 to 1.5 cm) to release the pus. The drainage should be cultured and examined with Gram's stain.

5

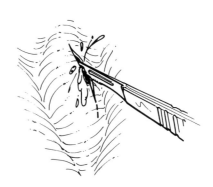

Insert a Malecot catheter and cut it to a length of 1 in. Transfix the projecting tube with a safety pin, and apply a dry, sterile dressing.

6

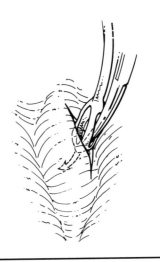

7

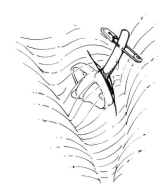

Leave the catheter in place for about two weeks, and then remove it by pulling the tubing up alongside a clamp in the same manner in which it was inserted. Antibiotics are probably not needed, but we usually prescribe a 5-day supply of a broad-spectrum drug. Most patients lose no time from work and complain of little discomfort except that they have to bathe more often. If they then follow the instructions given at the beginning of this chapter, they rarely have further difficulties.

RECURRENT PILONIDAL INFECTIONS

In spite of good hygiene, shaving, and hair removal, some patients continue to have repeated infections. In such patients marsupialization—the procedure described following—offers at least a 90% chance of permanent cure with little discomfort.

Carefully locate each of the pits or sinuses and excise these under lidocaine anesthesia with a small margin of skin so that all the openings are interconnected and laid open.

8

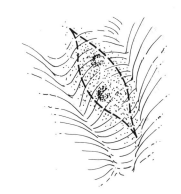

Very little of the skin need be removed. The object of the procedure is to unroof the sinus cavity and open all passages. Gently wipe the base with the end of the scalpel handle to get rid of resistant debris.

9

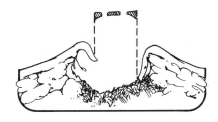

Loosely suture the edges of the incision to the base to minimize the granulating area.

10

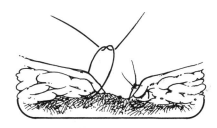

Sinuses are frequently found away from the midline. All these must be opened in a manner similar to that used for a midline pocket if further recurrences are to be avoided.

11

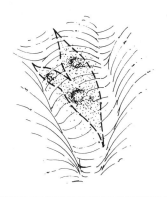

Most patients are able to return to their usual activities by the next day. We prescribe antibiotics for five days but are not convinced that these are necessary; the new Maxipads or similar adherent pads seem to be ideal and well tolerated. Healing takes about six weeks, but the wound appears to cause little difficulty in the patients' daily life.

Recurrences, although infrequent, are a possibility. When this happens, repeat the same procedure. The larger procedures sometimes recommended, such as the swinging of flaps, should be avoided. They do not carry a better success rate and are usually costly in terms of hospitalization, time lost from work, and patient discomfort.

24 · Selected Problems Affecting the Anus

WALTER J. PORIES, M.D.

HEMORRHOIDS

Hemorrhoids are a common affliction for which surgery is not often needed. These rectal varicosities can usually be controlled by increasing the proportion of fiber in the patient's diet, adding psyllium hydrophilic mucilloid (Metamucil) at 1 to 3 tablespoons per day to soften the stool, minimizing the time spent sitting on the toilet, avoiding straining, and occasionally using a soothing suppository such as Preparation H or Anusol. If the hemorrhoids are associated with bleeding, a sigmoidoscopy and, ideally, a barium enema should be performed to rule out other lesions. Too many cancers (and one is too many) have been missed because of the assumption that the patient's complaints were all due to hemorrhoids.

Evacuation of Thrombosed Hemorrhoids

Thrombosed hemorrhoids—swollen, intensely tender, and painful bluish masses that protrude from the anus—are easy to recognize. Because they are extremely tender, defer the rectal exam until the patient has recovered. The thrombosed hemorrhoid can be cured almost miraculously with an almost instantaneous relief of pain.

1

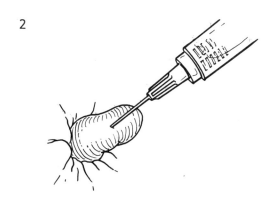

Gently inject the hemorrhoid with lidocaine and epinephrine through a #25 needle. The hemorrhoid is usually insensitive at its center because the mucosa at that point is usually ischemic from pressure. Patients are usually amazed that such a painful lesion can be treated without their feeling even the injection. If the injection is carried out in the right plane just under the mucosa (2 to 3 mm below the surface), the whole hemorrhoid turns white almost instantaneously and becomes insensitive.

2

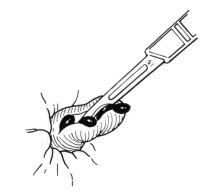

Make an incision of about 1 cm in the hemorrhoid. The incision must be quite deep because the edema usually thickens the mucosa and the clots are not encountered until the incision is about 0.5 cm or more in depth. The first clots surface almost spontaneously; the rest can usually be removed easily by forceps or gently milked from the anus with a finger in the rectum. The hemorrhoid shrinks quickly when it has been decompressed. Bleeding is rarely a problem and can easily be controlled by gentle pressure.

3

Insert a full tube of Nupercainal rectal ointment into the rectal canal through the applicator tip supplied with the tube. To empty the tube easily, grasp the base of the tube with a clamp and then wind the clamp in a manner similar to opening a sardine can.

4

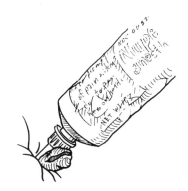

Relief is usually instantaneous. Patients are advised to soak in a bathtub two or three times over the first 24 hr and can usually return to their normal activities within one or two days.

Injection of Hemorrhoids

External hemorrhoids can be cured by the injection of thrombotic agents, a technique commonly used in the United Kingdom, rarely in the United States. The patient is placed in the lithotomy position as for a pelvic exam. If possible, the table is slightly tipped to elevate the head, causing the hemorrhoid to fill. The lesion is exposed through a slitted anoscope, injected with 0.5 ml of sodium morrhuate solution, and then compressed with the finger for 1 to 2 min. The hemorrhoid should thrombose within the hour. This process may be quite painful, and adequate analgesics should be prescribed.

Rubber-Band Ligature of Hemorrhoids

Rubber-band ligature of hemorrhoids has limited application because it can only be used for
hemorrhoids above the dentate line—the small
irregular line above which the anal mucosa becomes insensitive. Such isolated high hemorrhoids are rather unusual; most patients have
combined internal and external rectal varicosities. Unfortunately, the instrument is expensive,
and its limited application and its expense often
do not justify its purchase. It could, however,
be shared nicely among members of a group
of physicians.

5

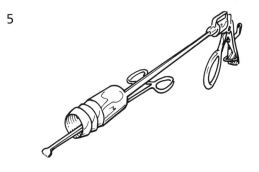

The banding procedure is convenient and safe
and can be performed through any well-illu-
minated proctoscope with a large lumen. The
banding instrument is tipped with a double tele-
scoping stainless-steel drum. To load the inner
drum, push tiny rubber bands (1/16-in diameter) up to the drum around a removable conical
tip. Release of rubber bands from the inner cylinder fires the instrument.

6

To carry out the banding, place the patient face
down in a flexed position. No anesthesia is
needed. Gently dilate the anus and introduce
the proctoscope. Then grasp the hemorrhoid at
its base with thin forceps that have been passed
through the inner cylinder of the banding instrument. If the patient has any discomfort, grasp
the hemorrhoid at a higher level—that is, several millimeters farther away from the dentate
line.

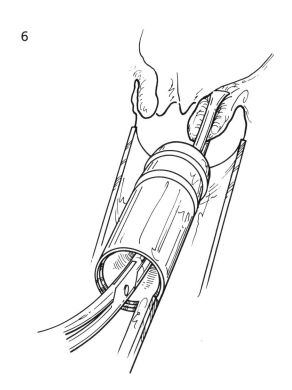

Next, pull the hemorrhoid snugly into the cylinder. Release the bands by closing the trigger. The banded hemorrhoid then becomes a bluish lump about 1 to 1.5 cm in diameter.

7

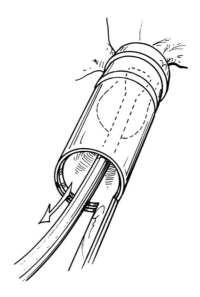

8

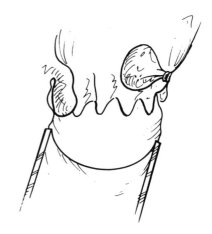

Band no more than two hemorrhoids at a time, and allow at least three weeks between bandings. The hemorrhoid will usually slough on the fourth to tenth day with a small amount of bleeding. Pain, though usually minimal or absent, can be a serious problem in a few patients for two to three days and may even require morphine. Caution patients about this possibility.

CONDYLOMATA ACUMINATA

Condylomata acuminata—soft, frondlike cutaneous polyps transmitted by sexual contact and probably caused by a virus—are most commonly seen on the vulva, anus, and penis. They are thought to be common in homosexual patients. Carefully screen individuals with such lesions for other venereal diseases.

Treat condylomata individually with local and *carefully limited* destruction of the individual lesions, avoiding injury to the normal skin. Two methods work well: cautery and the application of podophyllin. We prefer the cautery because the technique is more precise, but this method has the drawback of requiring anesthesia. In addition, severe strictures sometimes result from overzealous treatment of these lesions. Therefore, if the disease is extensive, divide the treatment into two or three sessions.

Cautery

Local anesthesia is required for the cautery technique. Infiltrate the base of each separate lesion or the area involving a mass of polyps with 1% lidocaine with epinephrine through a #25 needle. When the area is insensitive, lift each lesion with fine forceps or clamp and destroy it by touching that instrument *briefly* with the cautery. Do not allow burning to extend to normal skin.

9

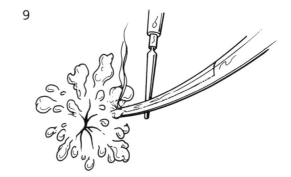

Application of Podophyllin

The application of tincture of podophyllin is easy
and painless. The technique requires careful
precision in limiting the podophyllin to the condylomata and avoiding any spill onto normal
skin. Anesthesia is not needed. Touch each con-
dyloma with a soaked Q-tip that has been fashioned to a fine point. Apply medication until
the lesions are clearly brown. Keep patient still
until the tincture has dried completely. A heat
lamp hastens the drying process.

The lesions usually slough in one or two weeks,
and the area heals within three weeks. Sitz baths
and the application of Nupercaine ointment can
help alleviate the discomfort of the posttreat-
ment period.

10

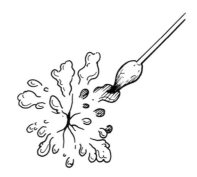

TREATMENT OF FISTULA IN ANO WITH A SETON

Fistula in ano, a common condition, results from
an earlier pararectal abscess that drained
through the skin. The tract is usually ragged
and narrowed by scars and therefore drains
poorly. Stool is occasionally expressed into the
tract during defecation, often occluding the
narrow passage. Therefore, repeated infections
with pain, fever, and bloody or purulent discharges frequently occur.

Goodsall's Rule is a useful guide for the local-
ization of the fistulous tracts: Fistulas that open
behind an imaginary line drawn through the
anus end in the posterior midline within the
anorectal canal; fistulas that open on the gen-
ital side of the line radiate like spokes of a
wheel. Anterior lesions are therefore usually easier to
thread than posterior fistulas.

11

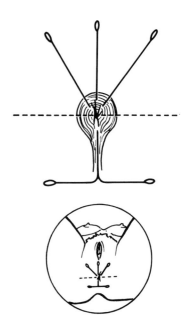

A fistula in ano should be excised if it is deep,
unroofed if superficial. Surgical procedures for
fistulas in ano are not well suited for office surgery because these operations are occasionally
technically difficult, painful, and associated with
considerable bleeding. Patients with fistulas are
best treated under general or spinal anesthesia
in a well-equipped operating room with adequate light and assistance.

12

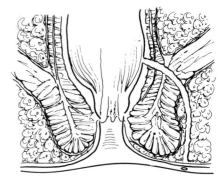

There are, however, instances when such an
operation is inappropriate because the patient
has other health problems or responsibilities. In
such cases, the seton tie provides a convenient
and safe approach that can be carried out in
the office. The seton tie, a heavy suture threaded

through the fistulous tract, serves as an indwelling drain that prevents blockage and abscess formation and as a technique for curing the condition by drawing the fistula out into the lumen of the anal canal.

Gently thread the fistula with a malleable silver probe carrying a #2 Marlex or similar nonabsorbable synthetic suture. Guide the probe by a finger within the anus. Threading the fistula with a seton tie may be difficult. Fistulas can have variable paths. They may run superficially just under the skin and mucosa, or they may wind their way deeply through or even outside the sphincter mechanism. Never force the probe because of the danger of making a false passage. Most failures of treatment with a seton tie are probably due to failure to thread the entire tract.

13
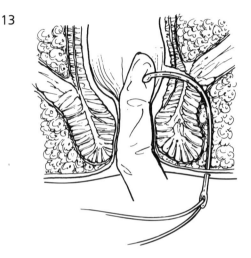

When the tip of the probe has progressed into the anal canal, bend the instrument into a ring and gently guide it out of the anus. Then tie the suture loosely but securely with at least five knots.

14
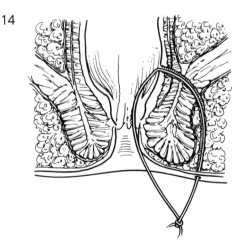

The suture will eventually work its way out of the tissues, drawing the fistula out and leaving behind a fine scar. The process can be compared to a thread cutting through an ice cube; the ice melts under the thread and freezes again behind it, thus preventing the cube from being cut in half.

15

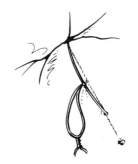

The process usually takes several weeks, but it may take months if the fistula is deep. It has the advantage of causing little discomfort, requires no time away from work, and almost always avoids the danger of incontinence.

Tightening the loop about once a week hastens the process. To accomplish this, tie another suture around the first loop. Avoid untying the initial loop because the seton tie can slip out easily, and rethreading it may be difficult, painful, and hard to justify to the patient.

The seton tie requires no special care. Instruct the patient to keep it clean by bathing frequently and using Tucks medicated rectal pads.

DRAINAGE OF PARARECTAL ABSCESSES

Pararectal abscesses are dangerous. These infections can spread rapidly into the ischiorectal space because the organisms are sometimes highly virulent, and delay is occasionally associated with septic portal vein phlebitis and metastatic abscesses. A red, tender area near the anus must be considered a pararectal abscess until proven otherwise. Use needle aspiration to diagnose and locate the pus pocket.

Infiltrate the tenderest area over the suspected abscess with 1% lidocaine and epinephrine. Insert a large-bore needle (at least a #18 because the pus may be thick and viscous) into the center of the suspected abscess, and aspirate the abscess with a 10-ml syringe. Do not withdraw the needle or aspirate all the pus because the abscess may be hard to find once it has been decompressed and the guiding needle has been removed.

16

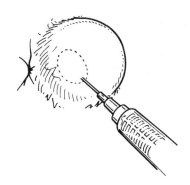

17

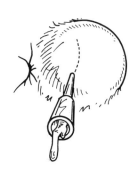

Incise the abscess with the needle as a guide. The incision should be generous enough to allow gentle introduction of a finger into the cavity. A 2- to 3-cm lesion will usually suffice. Have a large basin ready; a surprising amount of pus may often be obtained: 200 to 500 ml is not unusual.

18

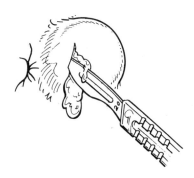

Place a Foley or Malecot catheter in the lesion for continuing drainage. If the incision is too large to retain one of these catheters, use Penrose drains that are marked with a safety pin and sewn in place. The patient should be treated heavily with a broad-spectrum antibiotic because many pararectal abscesses are due to mixed infections. Close follow-up is essential, especially in diabetic patients and others who are compromised by underlying diseases.

19

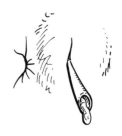

Examine the pus with Gram's stain (to guide antibiotic therapy), and culture it for aerobic and anaerobic organisms.

If the patient does not improve rapidly, poor drainage or inappropriate antibiotic coverage must be suspected. To appraise drainage, do a sinogram through the drainage tube and gently explore with a finger. Also, review the choice of antibiotics against the results from the bacteriology laboratory.

Urge patients to keep the area clean with frequent baths. Maxipads, which adhere to the patient's underclothing, make excellent dressings for drained pararectal abscesses. The drain can usually be removed after seven days, and healing can be expected in about three weeks.

25 · *Office Surgery of the Hands and Feet*

WALTER J. PORIES, M.D.

This chapter deals with those special problems of the hands and feet commonly seen in office practice, such as lesions of the nails, calluses, and infections. Please refer to Chapter 9 for the treatment of soft-tissue injuries and to Chapter 7 for the techniques for excision of small lesions.

The treatment of fractures and injuries of nerves, tendons, and vessels is beyond the scope of this book. An excellent and inexpensive reference for these and other complex surgical problems is *Handbook of Surgery* by T.S. Schrock (7th ed., Jones Medical Publications, Greenbrae, Calif., 1982).

SUBUNGUAL HEMATOMAS

Subungual hematomas are usually the result of a sudden blow or crush injury, such as the blow of a hammer or catching the fingertip in a car door. These collections of blood under the nail bed can be extremely painful yet can be relieved instantly and painlessly by draining the collection through a small hole in the nail. The hole can be made in two ways, by melting the nail with a paper clip or by boring the opening with a #11 scalpel blade.

For the first approach, heat the tip of a straightened paper clip with a match or cigarette lighter until it is red hot. Press the hot wire into the nail at the center of the hematoma until the dark blood escapes. Take care to warn the patient that the procedure is painless; the sight of a red-hot wire approaching an already painful finger is frightening. If the patient is unlikely to cooperate with the hot-paper-clip technique, use the more time-consuming method of boring a small hole with a #11 scalpel blade.

1

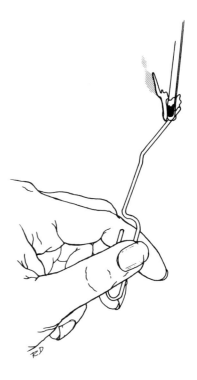

2

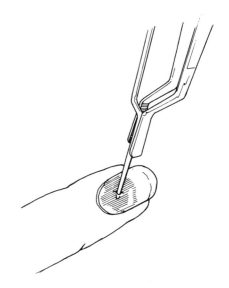

Relief is usually instantaneous, and a Band-aid usually suffices as a dressing. An X-ray examination of the finger should be done if a phalangeal or distal interphalangeal joint fracture is suspected.

INFECTIONS OF THE HANDS AND FINGERS

Infections of the hands are usually caused by trauma or retained foreign bodies such as splinters. Gram-positive cocci are the most commonly offending organisms, although other organisms such as *Clostridium tetani,* sporotrichosis, and fungi should be suspected if the infection does not respond rapidly to antibiotics, the involved area has an unusual appearance or manifests gangrene, or the patient's systemic manifestations appear unusually severe.

Most infections of the hands are superficial and respond rapidly to removal of the foreign body (if present) and application of a wet dressing. Antibiotics such as penicillin, erythromycin, or a cephalosporin should be given if there is more than a small margin of erythema, lymphangitis, lymphadenopathy, or fever.

PARONYCHIA

A paronychia is an abscess of the fingernail between the skin and the nail, usually caused by trauma and the entry of bacteria at the corner of the cuticle. Although many references advise incision of the abscess with a scalpel, such an approach is rarely if ever needed.

3

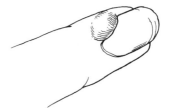

Soak the fingertip in soap and water for 15 to 20 min to soften the nail and cuticle. Gently and slowly push the softened cuticle laterally and proximally at the infected corner of the nail with a cotton swab until a drop of pus escapes from the abscess pocket. Persist in pushing until the pocket has been opened widely. Anesthesia is not needed, and the patient should have little discomfort.

4

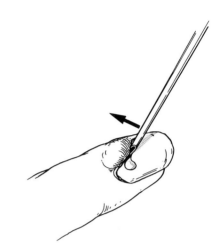

Apply an absorbent finger dressing (see Chapter 19) and instruct the patient to keep it moist. The paronychia will usually heal within 48 hr.

Antibiotics are rarely necessary, although persistent cases, such as those seen in fish handlers with streptococcal infection, may require a course of treatment with penicillin potassium.

A run-around is an advanced form of paronychia in which the pus has dissected around the entire base of the nail. The whole base of the nail is inflamed, and a large bubble of pus can usually be palpated under the nail.

5

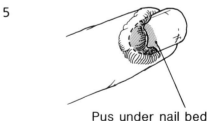

Pus under nail bed

It is not necessary to remove the entire nail to treat a run-around. Anesthesia is not required; if the procedure is gentle, there should be little discomfort.

Push the cuticle aside and away from the nail as described earlier. Continue the dissection until the pus begins to drain and the edge of the nail is visible. Insert one blade of an iris scissors under the nail, and transect the floating nail about 3 mm from its base.

6

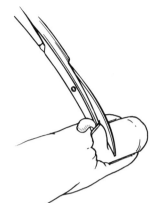

Lift the severed proximal portion of the nail out of its purulent bed, and apply a continuously moist finger dressing for about 48 hr.

7

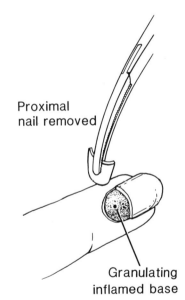

Proximal
nail removed

Granulating
inflamed base

The new nail will begin to grow back within four to six weeks. Leaving the distal portion of the nail in place provides comfort and a better appearance during the early period of repair.

SPACE INFECTIONS

Infections that extend into the subcutaneous fat of the fingers and the palm are called *space infections.* These are particularly dangerous because they progress rapidly, tunneling along tendon sheaths, and cause extensive tissue destruction. In a matter of hours such infections can produce long-standing or permanent disabilities. Fortunately, such infections are associated with considerable pain, which usually brings the patient to the doctor promptly. It is important to treat the infection immediately with adequate drainage, elevation, immobilization, and heavy doses of antibiotics.

Drainage of Space Infections

Infections of the deep spaces require wide drainage, but this must be accomplished without injury to the nerves, vessels, and complex tendinomuscular structures of the hand. In addition, incisions should be placed so that the scars do not cross any of the major tactile surfaces. A painful scar in any of these areas can seriously interfere with any manual activities, not only for those commonly called manual workers but also for those who use typewriters, play instruments, and punch cash registers. We all depend on our hands.

8

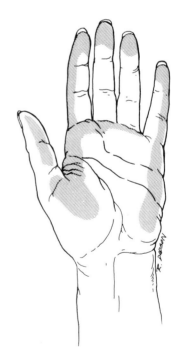

Incisions in the fingers and along each side of the hand should be made in a transverse plane. The neurovascular bundles are arranged at 45 degrees to this plane so that a lateral or medial incision into the digit can be carried to bone without danger of injuring the veins or vessels.

9

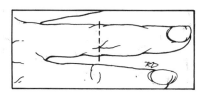

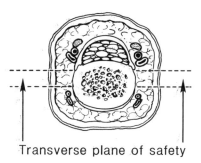

Transverse plane of safety

An excellent approach to locating the site of a safe incision is to draw a dot at the end of each of the creases at the interphalangeal and metacarpophalangeal joints. When the finger is straightened, these dots can be connected into a line of safety, which serves as the guide for incision and drainage.

10a

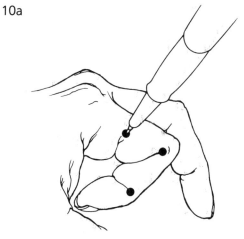

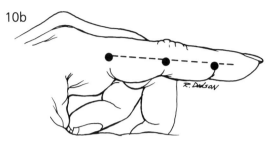

10b

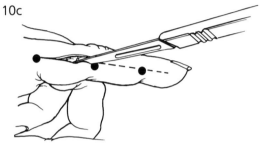

10c

If the diagnosis of a purulent collection is in doubt, aspirate the pulp. If you find pus, drainage should be done at once. Infiltrate the nontactile side of the finger with 1% lidocaine without epinephrine.

The proper placement of skin incisions into the fingers and hand is shown. In general, infections that require drainage of the deep spaces of the hand should be referred to a surgeon.

11

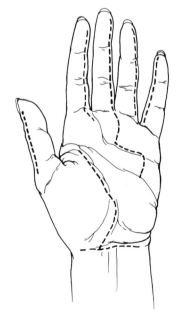

Felon

A felon is a space infection limited to the pulp of the fingertip. The swelling is sharply limited by the fascial boundaries of the space, both at the distal interphalangeal joint and within the radiating septa of the pulp space. Within hours of the onset of the infection, the fingertip becomes exquisitely painful from the ischemia produced by the increasing pressure of the infection. If the finger is not drained properly, the entire pulp and the future sensation and function of the fingertip may be lost.

12

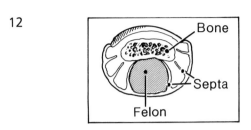

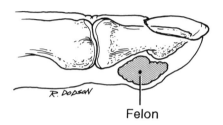

Felon

Drainage of a Felon

Incise along the line of safety deeply into the pulp of the finger until the pus is drained and there is an opening large enough for maintenance of adequate drainage (at least 1 cm long and 1 cm deep).

13

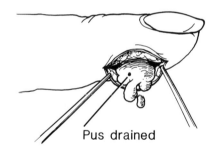

Pus drained

Insert a sterile rubber band, a small Penrose drain, or a strip of rubber cut from a sterile glove as a drain.

Dress the finger with a continuously moist dressing, splint and elevate the hand, and prescribe an antibiotic suitable against gram-positive infections. Provide prophylaxis against tetanus.

See the patient within 24 hr and change the dressing completely. If the condition of the patient and the wound is not clearly better, refer the case to a surgeon. Hand infections are serious and deserve a lot of respect.

FISHHOOK INJURIES

Fishhook injuries are common and are easily treated. Wash the fingertip with an antiseptic solution. Infiltrate the area around the tip of the fishhook with 1% lidocaine without epinephrine.

Advance the tip of the hook through the skin until the full barb protrudes.   14

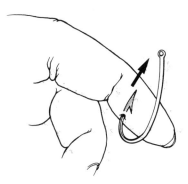

Cut the tip off the hook and withdrawn the now barbless shank.   15

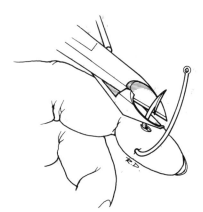

Another approach has been described, but we have had no personal experience with this method. Proponents claim that it can be done without anesthesia. Gently slide a #18 hypodermic needle along the shaft of the hook until the barb is engaged by the lumen of the needle. Then withdraw the hook.

16

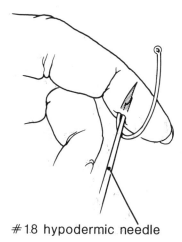

#18 hypodermic needle

INGROWN TOENAIL (UNGUIS INCARNATUS)

An ingrown toenail is caused by a spike of nail that remains after an improper trimming. The nail penetrates the soft tissue of the nailbed, producing an infection manifested by increasing pain on walking and foul-smelling granulations. Treatment consists in cutting off the offending spike and educating the patient in proper nail care.

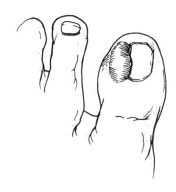

Soak the foot for 15 to 20 min in soapy water to cleanse the area and soften the nail. No anesthesia is necessary if the procedure is done gently and patiently.

Elevate the edge of the nail out of its bed by
gently pushing small bits of cotton, 2 × 3 mm
in size, under the nail until the edge of the nail
and the spike are visible.

18

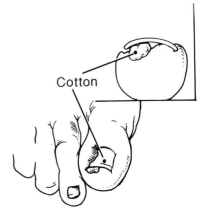

Cotton

Trim the nail to a smooth edge with an iris
scissors.

19

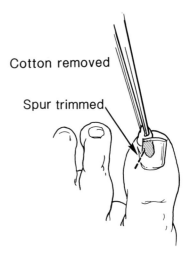

Cotton removed

Spur trimmed

Remove the cotton from beneath the nail. The
relief of pain is usually dramatic. A dressing is
not normally required.

Instruct the patient to bathe the foot regularly
until healing is complete, usually in three to four
days.

Instruct the patient how to cut the nail so that the condition will not recur. The nail should be cut in a straight rather than a curved line, preferably with a toenail clipper rather than a scissors.

20

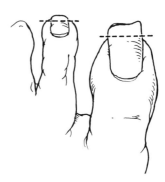

PLANTAR WART

Plantar warts are hard, calluslike, concentric collections of keratin, which act like a stone in a shoe, making walking increasingly painful. Plantar warts are difficult, if not impossible, to cure. Radical excision of the lesion with an oval of skin is not justified because the procedure is often followed by recurrence in another part of the foot and often leaves a painful scar.

21

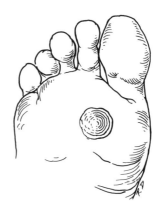

Three approaches are used today: (1) abrasion with an emery board (time consuming, but safe); (2) use of a keratolytic agent to soften and dissolve the lesion (medicated foot pads are available for this purpose from drugstores; a crushed moistened aspirin in a Band-aid is an effective substitute); and (3) excision of the central keratin core, which can be done easily and painlessly, giving immediate relief.

Soak the foot in soapy water for 15 to 20 min
to soften the keratin. Examine the lesion carefully and find the fine line of cleavage between
the keratin ball and the outer ring of the plantar
wart. No anesthetic is needed. The procedure
should be painless.

Incise this circular border with an iris scissors.   22
A line of cleavage will develop easily.

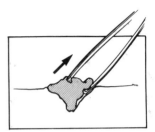

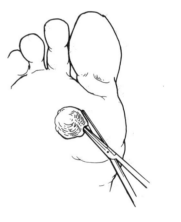

Lift the keratin ball out of its bed by gently
following the line of cleavage. Occasionally, the
patient may feel a brief twinge as the deepest
point of attachment is severed.

No dressing is needed. The patient can be allowed to walk at once.

Occasionally, plantar warts can be kept under
better control by fitting the patient with different shoes. We have not found this helpful and

consider it an unnecessary expense. In most cases, the patient or the family can be instructed in the control of plantar warts. Young, intelligent patients with good eyesight can be taught to remove the lesions with a fine pair of scissors; older patients with infirmities do better with medicated foot pads and an emery board.

CORNS

Corns are calluses that form as a result of pressure from poorly fitting shoes; they are especially common if the toes are deformed or if there are bunions. Corns are best treated by the fitting of looser shoes and the application of medicated corn pads, various-sized self-adhesive bandages impregnated with a keratolytic agent.

If the corns have become so painful that something must be done at once rather than waiting for the slow action of a corn plaster, the corn can be trimmed.

Examine the foot carefully to rule out underlying vascular disease before undertaking to trim the corn. An ischemic foot may not heal, and the excision of the corn may be blamed for the subsequently required amputation.

Soak the foot in soapy water for 15 to 20 min to soften the corn. Paint the toe with an antiseptic solution.

Trim the corn, in layers, from the top down, with a pair of iris scissors until a relatively normal contour of the toe is achieved. No dressing is needed.

Instruct the patient to be fitted with shoes that do not compress the toes and to treat the remaining corn with a corn plaster.

CARE OF THE FEET IN DIABETIC PATIENTS

Good foot care can prevent many amputations in diabetic patients, especially those who have good peripheral circulation in neuropathic feet.

Diabetes is a cruel disease. Diabetic patients heal poorly, have little resistance to infection, have decreased sensation in areas most vulnerable to trauma, and often have only marginal vision. They can't see the tack on the floor, can't feel it when they step on it, and have little resistance to the infection that follows. If they try to inspect their feet, their vision is inadequate to let them see the lesions.

A good approach to diabetic foot care is to instruct the family to examine the foot weekly and to return to the doctor for a monthly inspection. During these monthly visits several particulars should be dealt with. Trim the nails with a large nail clipper straight across at the end of each toe. Trim any calluses and plantar warts as previously described. If there are large thick sheets of keratin, soak the foot to soften them, and trim them flush.

Examine the spaces between the toes for moisture, gangrene, and breaks in the skin. If any of these is present, instruct the family to apply rubbing alcohol liberally four times a day, let it evaporate to dryness, and then keep the toes apart with pledgets of cotton.

Examine the foot carefully, especially the heel and the toes, for areas of discoloration and gangrene. Palpate for the dorsalis pedis and posterior tibial pulses; if these cannot be detected, the patient may benefit from a consultation with a vascular surgeon and quantification of the circulation in a noninvasive vascular laboratory.

GANGRENE OF THE TOES

Gangrene of the toes, an ominous sign of ischemia, calls for thorough study by a vascular surgeon to evaluate the need for immediate emergency surgery and the potential for vascular reconstruction.

Some patients will not be candidates for surgery, however, while others, in spite of surgery, will be left with one or several gangrenous digits. These are often treated in the family physician's office.

23 The most important principle to remember is that dry gangrene is well tolerated, wet gangrene is dangerous. Dry gangrene is truly dry. The tissues are coal black, dry, and free of odor and pain. In contrast, wet gangrene has a brownish cast with some maceration in the crevices. In addition, the area around the wet gangrene is often painful and red.

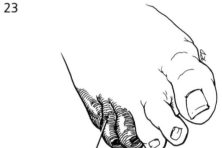

Dry gangrene

Dry Gangrene

24 Instruct the patient to wash the gangrenous area four times a day with a pledget of cotton soaked with rubbing alcohol.

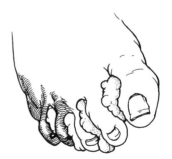

The surfaces should be allowed to dry fully and then padded between the toes with cotton.

25

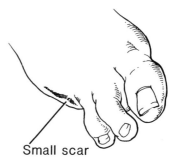

Small scar

The limb should be used normally. The patient should be encouraged to walk on the dead toe or toes.

The gangrenous portion will demarcate and separate spontaneously in about two to three months, leaving a well-healed scar. Prepare the patient and the family for this event, and instruct them to bring the separated digits to you for disposal.

When gangrene is present, follow the patient closely, with visits once a week or so, to be certain that the gangrene remains dry and does not advance.

Wet Gangrene

Small areas of moisture may still be amenable to office treatment. Begin broad-spectrum antibiotic therapy, being certain that your instructions regarding alcohol dehydration and cotton separations are carefully followed, and see the patient daily. If the process does not show prompt signs of improvement, the patient needs immediate hospitalization for IV antibiotic therapy, possible drainage, and perhaps even amputation.

STASIS DERMATITIS AND VENOUS ULCERS

Stasis ulcers are a common consequence of deep venous disease. In the normal limb, valves in the superficial and deep veins direct the flow of blood toward the heart. The blood is pumped by the contraction of leg muscles within the rigid fascial envelopes.

Phlebitis destroys the venous valves, rendering the venous pump ineffective. The venous blood thus puddles in the area, preventing oxygenated arterial blood with nutrients fron entering the extrafascial tissues of the lower leg. The skin, ischemic and malnourished, becomes discolored with hemosiderin, scarred, and vulnerable to injury. Because the area above the medial malleolus is most vulnerable, it breaks down first, but eventually a severe stasis ulcer can involve the entire circumference of the lower leg.

Therapy is directed toward compressing the surficial and perforating veins so that the unoxygenated blood cannot puddle in the cutaneous vessels but is instead directed proximally through the muscular pump.

Examine the extremity carefully to be certain that there is no evidence of arterial or lymphatic disease. Most patients with stasis disease demonstrate large varicose veins and thick woody induration and discoloration about the ankles, most severe on the medial surface. The leg is usually edematous, and the skin flakes readily. If an ulcer is present, it is usually just proximal to the medial malleolus.

If the chief complaint is pain and the skin is intact, fit a heavy elastic stocking to the leg. For most patients, the stockings sold by Sears are reasonable in cost and serve well; for patients with large legs or severe disease, individually

26

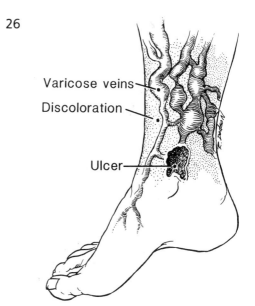

Varicose veins

Discoloration

Ulcer

fitted stockings from a company such as Jobst may be needed.

Elastic stockings are expensive and require careful handling if they are to last. Instruct your patients to wash them daily in cold water with a gentle cold-water soap, such as Woolite. Elastic hose slip on far more easily if the patient wears an old nylon stocking underneath.

Avoid roll-type elastic bandages for the treatment of venous disease. They are difficult to apply, rarely stay in place, and tend to bunch up to form tourniquets which impede rather than promote venous drainage.

Most patients with stasis disease consult the physician only after they have an ulcer. By then the pain is often so severe that they fear they need an amputation. Most such cases, no matter how severe the ulcer, can be treated on an outpatient basis. Wash the ulcer gently with soap and water, then apply an Unna paste boot (Dohme's paste) as described in Chapter 18. Most patients feel better within 24 hr, and healing is usually evident within two weeks. The boot needs to be reapplied weekly. When healing is complete, usually after two to three months, switch the patient from the Unna boot to heavy elastic stockings.

Some patients with stasis disease can benefit and even be cured by surgery. In a few cases where the stasis is due to a localized occlusion of one iliac vein, a bypass graft to the patent side can produce remarkable results. Others may benefit from a Linton procedure, an operation directed toward the ligation and interruption of the incompetent perforating veins of the lower leg. Accordingly, in difficult or long-standing cases of deep venous disease, secure consultation with a vascular surgeon.

Index